ADVANCING NURSING
EDUCATION WORLDWIDE

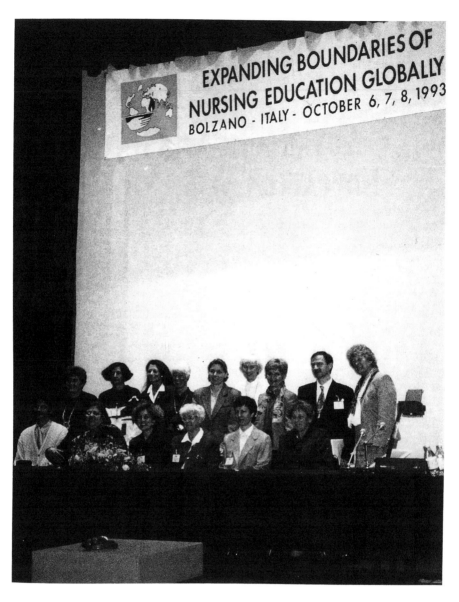

Frontispiece: Scientific Committee of the Bolzano Conference.

Advancing Nursing Education Worldwide

Doris M. Modly, RN, PhD, and
Joyce J. Fitzpatrick, RN, PhD, FAAN,
both of Case Western Reserve University

and

Piera Poletti and Renzo Zanotti, IP, AFD, PhD,
both of CEREF and the International Institute of Nursing
Research in Padua, Italy

Editors

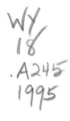

 Springer Publishing Company

Copyright © 1995 by Springer Publishing Company, Inc.

Springer Publishing Company, Inc.
536 Broadway
New York, NY 10012

Cover design by Tom Yabut
Production Editor: Joyce Noulas
Cover art by Isabella Nebl

95 96 97 98 99 / 5 4 3 2 1

Library of Congress Cataloging-in-Publication Data

Advancing nursing education worldwide / Doris Modly . . . [et al.]
    editors.
        p. cm.
    Includes bibliographical references and index.
    ISBN 0–8261–8650–5
    1. Nursing—Study and teaching—Congresses. 2. Nursing—Study and teaching—International cooperation—Congresses. I. Modly, Doris Matherny.
    RT73.A36 1994
    610.73\071\1—dc20   94–35282
                                                                            CIP

Printed in the United States of America

Contents

Contributors

Margaret F. Alexander, RGN, SCM, RNT, BSC, PhD, FRCN
Professor and Head of Department of Health & Nursing Studies
Glasgow, Caledonia University
Glasgow, Scotland, UK

Irmajean Bajnok, RN, PhD
Program Director of Nursing-International, Director WHO Collaborating Center
Mount Sinai Hospital
Toronto, ON, Canada

Colleen Conway-Welch, RN, PhD, CNM, FAAN
Dean School of Nursing
Vanderbilt University
Nashville, TN

Joyce J. Fitzpatrick, RN, MBA, PhD, FAAN
Professor and Dean of Nursing
Case Western Reserve University
Cleveland, OH

Kornelia K. Helembai, RN, PhD
Head of Department of Nursing
College of Health Sciences
Albert Szertgyorgyi Medical University
Szeged, Hungary

Magister Brigitta Hochenegger-Haubmann
School of Nursing
Leoben, Austria

Zeinab Loutfi, RN, PhD
Director of High Institute of Nursing
Ain-Shams University
Cairo, Egypt

Geraldine McCarthy, RGN, RNT, MED, MSN, PhD
College Lecturer-Nursing Studies
University College
Cork, Ireland

Diane McGivern, RN, PhD, FAAN
Head New York University Division of Nursing
New York, NY

Mary O. Mundinger, RN, PhD, FAAN
Dean, Columbia University School of Nursing
New York, NY

Doris M. Modly, RN, MA, PhD
Associate Professor
Director, International Health
   Program and World Health
   Organization Collaborating
   Center for Nursing
Case Western Reserve University
Cleveland, OH

Dott. Piera Poletti
Director of CEREF, Center of
   Nursing Research and Education
Padua, Italy

Sheila A. Ryan, RN, PhD, FAAN
Dean School of Nursing
University of Rochester
Rochester, NY

Jane Salvage, RN, BA, MSC
Regional Advisor for Nursing and
   Midwifery, WHO Europe
Copenhagen, Denmark

Majda Slajmer-Japelj, RN, Soc.
International Manager, WHO
   Collaborative Centre
Maribor, Slovenia

Ursula Springer, PhD
Springer Publishing Company, Inc.
New York, NY

Marta Stankova, PhD
Professor of Theory and Practice of
   Nursing
Charles University
Prague, Czech Republic

Marianne Tallberg, RN, PhD
Associate Professor
Helsingfors, Finland

Renzo Zanotti, IP, AFD, PhD
Director of ISIRI, International
   Institute of Nursing Research
Padua, Italy

Preface

This book presents the key papers of the first international conference on Nursing Education, "Expanding Boundaries of Nursing Education Globally: Focus on Nursing Education Research," held in Bolzano, Italy, in October of 1993. Nurse Educators from 36 countries attended. The conference was organized by ISIRI International Institute of Nursing Research (Padua, Italy), Case Western Reserve University (Cleveland, Ohio), and Autonomous Province Bozen, Health Councillor and Province Board of Nursing (Bozen, Italy). Additional supporters from the United States included Schools of Nursing from the following universities: Columbia, New York, Rochester, and Vanderbilt, and from Italy, the University of Padua. The conference was designed to provide an opportunity for nurse teachers, leaders, and scientists to share their education and research experiences and identify perspectives for the future. The time seemed to be right because of the dramatic changes going on in nursing educational systems throughout the world. In many countries basic nursing education recently has been undergoing much revision. In many countries the system of nursing education is moving from hospital-based to university-based schools, and professional education in general is being upgraded.

The conference purposes were to provide an opportunity for international nursing leaders to share innovative approaches to nursing education toward the goals of:

1. Expanding the boundaries of nursing education worldwide;
2. Sharing innovative approaches to nursing education, including faculty and student exchange programs;
3. Reporting cross-cultural and collaborative research;
4. Developing collaborative research.

The aim of this book is to provide for a wider dissemination of the information shared at the conference.

The conference was planned through a Scientific Committee comprised of an international group of nursing leaders. The members met to choose the papers to be presented at the conference but also to develop a strategic document to use as a manifesto to draw the nursing community's attention to the need for increasing nursing education research. The document is presented here as the final chapter of this book. In order to fulfill the conference mission it must be widely distributed in as many countries as possible. Therefore, we hope readers will request permission to reproduce it for colleagues and students in journals, books, and school materials, and use it as a stimulus for discussion to develop new research projects. Many targeted research areas are suggested, as are strategies for funding.

The topics presented in this book were chosen based on the most important areas of advancements in nursing education. In the editors' view, nursing education research has to be like a puzzle, where the structure is already drawn, but pieces have still to be included, through additional experience and research. This book forms the beginning outline of the puzzle.

In the first chapter Salvage presents a broad picture of global trends in the education of nurses. The issues are discussed from the perspective of health development, which is the World Health Organization's mission. Salvage provides a framework for exploring how education can help to improve the health of individuals and communities.

In the second chapter Modly and Springer summarize patterns of nursing education requirements worldwide. This chapter was developed specifically for this book, after the conference.

In the following chapter, Zanotti explores the potentials of education and research in broadening nursing boundaries, from the discipline and the profession's points of view. His presentation sets the stage for the rest of the book by stressing the importance of implementing programs that go beyond the boundaries of a specific country's culture.

Mundinger presents changes going on in nurses' functions in the United States' health services and discusses implications for professional practice and nursing education at national and international levels.

In Chapter 5, Modly presents factors to be considered in the process of curriculum construction and implementation to meet present practice requirements and develop future practice. Modly analyzes curriculum context's impact, introducing examples from the United States and East Europe.

In Chapter 6, McCarthy describes the results of research on teaching methods in nursing, considering the learning process, methods' effectiveness and efficiency, and students' satisfaction.

Hochenegger-Haubmann discusses the evolution of nursing education and its implications for practice and teaching. She stresses the peculiarity of nursing preparation and teachers' roles in carrying out the educational tasks.

The importance of teaching research at every level of education is stressed in the following chapter by Poletti. Referring to nursing literature, she describes strategies and methods introduced to teach research. A scenario for further development is provided.

One of the most compelling topics in nursing education is the integration between theoretical and clinical teaching. A thorough examination of the topic is reported by Alexander, who describes the state of the art, but also poses questions for the future.

Two different approaches to teaching clinical judgment are introduced by Stankova in Chapter 10, referring to the learning process and the contextual working culture. Research findings are included to support the author's assumptions.

As the change in education has to refer to a model assumed by the community and the professional group as one suitable for the health demands, Slajmer-Japelj introduces and analyzes key issues in developing a new model for nursing education.

The education process has to provide students with the competencies they will require in carrying out their role. However, sometimes it fails in helping students to develop their own professional identity. To learn attitudes and not just knowledge and skills is the cutting edge in nursing students' preparation. Helembai focuses her contribution on this key issue in Chapter 12.

Loutfi underlines the necessity to consider attitude development in nursing curricula with particular attention to the development of ethical components. In Chapter 13, she explains the reasons for an increase in attention to the topic and provides information on how to include ethical content in nursing programs.

Managerial roles will assume more and more importance in the health services at every level in all countries. An analysis of the development in the United States of America is presented in Chapter 14 by Ryan and Conway-Welch.

Computers can be used widely in nursing education for many purposes, described in Chapter 15. Tallberg warns about the underuse of computers and introduces some instructions to prepare students to use them.

In the last few years the phenomenon of re-entry in job position has been assuming a bigger dimension in many countries. As a consequence, basic and continuing education programs have had to take into account adult learning. McGivern describes many aspects of the argument in Chapter 16.

Bajnok presents a model for understanding the organizational aspects of nursing education from the perspectives of social, political, economic, technical, and cultural realities specific to each country in Chapter 17.

Fitzpatrick describes roles and responsibilities of nurses at different levels and positions in implementing nursing education research toward a global interaction.

We hope this book will provide the reader with a broad view of the status and the trends in research on nursing education worldwide. It should be useful to professional policymakers, deans and directors of nursing schools, teachers and doctoral students in nursing and education. International cooperation was a goal of the conference and the book includes contributions of authors from 12 countries. It is perhaps the first to use this approach and we hope many will follow. A purpose of the book is to stimulate the development of research on education globally; some authors chose to describe their country's experience, others have tried to introduce a more global approach. In fact, it is not easy to have a world perspective for many reasons; perhaps the most important being the difficulty of many people to communicate in English. As a consequence, most experiences are communicated just at the national level, and data are therefore difficult to collect. An increase in exchanging information and knowledge is an important aim for the nursing community and this book could be a stimulus.

We hope this is the first of a series of books on this subject and other topics in nursing produced with a worldwide perspective—the approach of the future. We like to imagine this book as a sower and hope to see its products brought to the second conference aimed to expand the boundaries of nursing education globally.

THE EDITORS

PART I

Overview

CHAPTER 1

Global Trends in Nursing Education: A World Health Organization Perspective

Jane Salvage, RN, BA, MSC

I mproving the quality of the basic and continuing education of nurses and midwives has never been more important than it is today. In all countries of the world, rich or poor, industrial or rural, people doing nursing work are by far the largest group employed in health services—so the effectiveness or otherwise of nursing and midwifery interventions must inevitably be a key influence on health. While there is still much work to be done on establishing the precise nature of the link between educational input and health outcomes, no one doubts that in general, the better educated the professional, the more likely they are to perform well and to contribute to health gain. That contribution has never been more needed than it is today.

This Chapter presents a broad picture of global trends in the education of nurses, midwives, and related health professionals. (The titles of these professional categories vary from country to country, and may include feldschers, health visitors, paramedics and others; hereafter they will all be referred to simply as "nurses" for brevity.) The issues are discussed from the perspective of health development rather than professionalization: in other words, the starting point is WHO's mission to work towards the goal of health for all. That mission provides a framework for exploring how education can help to improve the health of individuals and communities. The development of nursing as a profession, on the other hand, is an important but secondary concern.

First, a description of the global health situation today, and an assessment of how nursing is responding to the challenges is presented. A brief description is given of WHO policies and activities in nursing education worldwide, and a summary of some common concerns in the future development of education. Nursing reform in the countries of Central and Eastern Europe and the former USSR will be highlighted—which raises questions about how to ensure that international cooperation in nursing education is appropriate and useful.

THE GLOBAL HEALTH PICTURE

The education of health professionals is not an end in itself, but a means to help people achieve better health, a better quality of life, or a dignified death.

Education programs which are divorced from the immediate needs of the target population are a luxury which few, if any, countries can afford in these times of global economic recession. This is not to argue that academic institutions, that is, those with a theoretical and research bias, have no contribution to make, for there is nothing as practical as good theory. However, the goal of better health must be kept firmly in mind at all times, even in an ivory tower. Designing effective, outcome-oriented programs must begin with an assessment of today's health needs—and tomorrow's health trends, since the programs will prepare practitioners for the future as well as for now.

What can be said about the global picture, bearing in mind that every country, region, and even village has its own unique characteristics, strengths, and needs? The variety is, of course, enormous. One indicator is the relative amounts spent on health care. Overall, about 8% of the world's total income is spent on health care, but that ranges from less than $10 to more than $2700 per person from country to country. Generalizations about global health are therefore difficult to make. A succinct overview was recently provided by the WHO Headquarters Study Group on Nursing Beyond the Year 2000, which summarized the key global health issues as population growth and demographic transitions; infectious and parasitic diseases; and health-related vulnerability (World Health Organization [WHO], 1993a).

Population growth is still a major obstacle to health for all despite the slowing down which has occurred since 1970. One in three of the world's population is now aged between 10 and 24, raising the prospect of even greater growth in future. In developing regions the urban population is projected to triple in the next 30 years, which will have a huge impact on patterns of health and health care. Meanwhile the deceleration in population growth, accompanied by remarkable gains in life expectancy, has increased the proportion of old people, bringing greater needs for social support for the well elderly and care for those with chronic health needs. Ironically, too, increased affluence has exacerbated the long-term problems of mental illness, heart disease, cancer, and alcohol-related diseases in many countries.

The second major issue identified by the Study Group is infectious and parasitic diseases, which continue to have devastating effects, especially on the poor. Immunization programs have brought success, but poliomyelitis, measles, whooping cough, and neonatal tetanus are still major killers. Cholera, leprosy, and tuberculosis continue to result in avoidable deaths and disabilities; malaria is worsening in many places; and AIDS still poses a major threat to global health.

A person's health is influenced by a complex array of cultural, political, and socioeconomic factors. Various forms of social and economic deprivation, acting simultaneously, create health-related vulnerability, which is reflected in patterns of fertility, illness, and death. The most vulnerable groups include women, children, the frail elderly, and those who are not economically productive. To take only two examples, a woman in sub-Saharan Africa who becomes pregnant is 75 times more likely to die as a result than a woman in western Europe (World Bank, 1993). Meanwhile, a third of all children in developing countries suffer from malnutrition.

Describing these problems may have limited impact, now that we have become so used to seeing images of death and suffering on television or in the newspapers, and perhaps have become hardened to them. The examples also may seem rather remote to those of us fortunate enough to live or work in richer countries—though complacency in unwise, as recent events in Europe have demonstrated. Yet, although such problems are distant from the educationist's daily business of curriculum review or seminar preparation, they are the foundation stone of the education debate. Huge inequalities in health exist within as well as between countries, and we must focus ever more clearly on how nurses in every country can improve the health of groups at risk, because that is where the major health needs lie. The challenge to educationists, and to the rest of us, is to devise education programs which equip nurses to meet that challenge effectively.

Against this backdrop of continuing challenges to health, the Study Group found, there is increasing inequity in income distribution and access to health care. The vulnerable are becoming more vulnerable, and growing poverty in many countries is reflected in worsening health. Previous gains in health and health care are being lost as costs rise and resources shrink. Meeting the health needs of the future will require careful use of resources, and making health care interventions where they can have the most impact—which will require less hierarchical, more flexible, multidisciplinary, and multisectoral health care systems.

Nurses must therefore be prepared to reorient practice and therefore education to meet changing needs, and to work more closely with service users, informal carers, and other health personnel. Health care needs and the factors influencing health will be complex, multifaceted, and changeable, and health care systems will look radically different in future. According to the Study Group it is critical for WHO and countries to look toward these future developments and begin the process of change immediately and to recognize the need for ongoing review and evaluation so as to respond rapidly to change.

THE RESPONSE OF NURSES AND MIDWIVES

How have nurses responded to these challenges to date? Despite their relatively low status and lack of formal power (or perhaps, in some ways, because of it, giving them fewer vested interests to defend), the reaction has been heartening. It is recognized everywhere that professional practice must be more finely tuned to meet priority needs, and that a major shift is needed away from the role of servant to the medical profession, towards the role of helper and partner of people and communities. In my work with WHO I meet nurses from all parts of the world, it has been surprising how widely our perceptions and aspirations are shared from one region to another. The need for a new nursing role, and therefore the need for education reform, is mentioned everywhere.

WHO has taken these issues to heart, as shown in the work of the Study Group described above. The Group's report will be published and will contain important recommendations to WHO and to countries, based on three main strategic thrusts. These are: the need for a new multisectoral approach to health care; a shift in the focus of workforce development in nursing to reflect the health needs of countries; and revitalization and reorientation of nursing education and practice to meet the challenges of the future.

Several of the recommendations make special reference to nursing education, as follows:

- WHO and countries should continue to support the development of innovative, cost-effective nursing and midwifery educational programs which are focused on the development of critical thinking and a caring attitude. In particular, WHO should support management training, and the development and use of relevant learning materials.
- Countries should ensure that students entering nursing and midwifery programs have a good basic education and have reached a level of maturity consistent with the responsibilities of the work.
- In deciding on the appropriateness of basic and postbasic education in nursing at the university level, countries should consider:

  - future health care needs and the roles of nurses and midwives;
  - the level of general education in the country; and
  - the educational patterns of other professions in the health care field.

  When appropriate, countries should move basic nursing education to the university.

- Countries should ensure that basic and continuing nursing and midwifery education are focused on knowledge and skills that are relevant to, and attitudes that are respectful of, the needs and values of local communities, and that innovations which are produced through continuing education become part of basic professional education.

These recommendations, and the others produced by the Study Group, will be introduced into the debates of another important international committee, the WHO Global Advisory Group on Nursing and Midwifery. This Group was established in 1992 at the request of the World Health Assembly, WHO's global parliament, to accelerate progress in nursing development—in response to widespread recognition that many factors still obstruct the effective delivery of nursing services around the world. As WHO's Director General wrote to the health ministers of all Member States in April 1993, these factors include the shortage of nurses and midwives in terms of service needs, the problems of inadequate material support for nurses and midwives, and the lack of input by nurses and midwives at the policy level. Although these problems were not new, the Director General said, little progress had been made towards solving them.

The work of the Global Advisory Group continues and it met in November 1993. It identified as a major issue in its first report (WHO, 1993b) the need to address basic, postbasic, and continuing education needs in nursing. Similar concerns and similar goals also were very much in evidence at the recent quadrennial congresses of the International Council of Nurses and the International Confederation of Midwives. Globally, then, nursing leaders are acutely aware of the need for radical change in nursing and the corresponding need for reform of nursing education at all levels. This strategic and, hopefully, united effort at the global level will provide essential support and stimulation for regions and countries to address the issues.

A review of nursing education activities being carried out in the six WHO regions reveals a similar preoccupation with change. Despite repeated complaints of the lack of resources for nursing development, projects are under way in every region: some of the countries which are working closely with their WHO Regional Office on nursing education are Bahrain, Bangladesh, Congo, Ecuador, Hungary, India, Indonesia, Kazakhstan, Laos, Lithuania, the Maldives, Mexico, Myanmar, Nepal, Nicaragua, Panama, Papua New Guinea, Qatar, Romania, Slovenia, Sri Lanka, Tonga, and Zambia. Nursing education change is a global concern. There is also remarkable similarity in the issues being tackled, primarily curriculum review and reorientation to primary health care at all levels of the educational systems; new program development, especially in higher education; training of nurse teachers; provision of good-quality learning materials; continuing education schemes; closer links between education and service; and, perhaps a more recent trend, the evaluation of outcomes.

This list of activities is in any case only the tip of the iceberg. In many if not most countries, a myriad of similar projects is under way, organized by ministries of health and education, health authorities, universities, professional associations, and voluntary organizations. Amid this great variety, it is possible to trace some common concerns. Above all, there are growing efforts to strengthen the relationship between health need, health policy, and the education of health professionals. All too often in the past, and still today, there has been inadequate linkage between these issues: health/health care policy is based more on political considerations, professional demands, and historical precedents than on analysis of what would make most impact on health. Then again, health policy is too seldom reflected in educational programs, when it should be the driving force, ensuring that professionals are trained to acquire the competencies needed to turn visions and policies into practical action.

The search for cost-effectiveness often provides the spur for this clearer thinking. No country can now afford, if it ever could, the luxury of training health professionals whose work makes no impact on health and health care, and whose practice may even be harmful. The results of nursing practice are being scrutinized more closely than ever before, within the profession but also by the economists; we are now obliged to demonstrate our value, and our value for money, by measuring the outcomes of nursing intervention. This is difficult, especially as the resources to undertake such evaluation are in short supply, and so many of the beneficial effects of nursing are difficult, maybe impossible, to measure. Yet nurses have little option if they wish to see the profession flourish in this tough environment.

This in turn poses a special challenge to nursing educationists, who must work more closely than ever before with policy-makers and service providers to ensure that the student practitioner acquires the appropriate competencies, skill, and knowledge. It is increasingly recognized that old norms, such as the length of training and the ratio of clinical to classroom education, are inadequate indicators of educational quality, and that the success of a program must instead be judged by its outcomes. For example, national and international bodies often insist that basic nursing education should be 4600 hours long—but if the quality and outcome of such a program is not measured, who is to say this is a better use of society's resources than a program lasting only two years? We need to define realistic indicators of progress in nursing education development which go beyond these crude old norms. It is a complex task, but the only way forward—and it will be impossible without close cooperation between nursing leaders, service providers, educationists, and experts in education research.

A third international concern is centered on the position of nursing in society and its public image. The public still perceives nursing as a necessary but low-status occupation for which minimal training is required. Nurses are supposed to be born, not made, and the essential requirements of a good nurse are a nice personality and a strong pair of feet. The idea that nursing education should have the status of a university degree is alien to most people. Such attitudes prevail in medical and policy-making circles too, and although they are changing, they are not changing fast enough. The other side of this double bind is the continuing domination of health services by the medical model of health and illness, with its tendency to undervalue humanistic, psychosocial care in favor of disease-based technological interventions—put another way, the ascendancy of masculine over feminine values.

NURSING REFORM IN CENTRAL AND EASTERN EUROPE

These concerns, which are shared by nurses from all parts of the globe, are especially salient for countries undertaking major nursing reforms. In WHO's European Region, a nursing renaissance is beginning in many of the countries whose health care systems were based on the Soviet model. While this had many strengths, not least in providing universal access to health care, it neglected nursing shamefully. Caring was simply not valued; the connection between feeling better and getting better was not understood; and health care was primarily medical, disease-based, and technocratic. Now, at this time of crisis and opportunity, countries whose nursing traditions decayed, or where nursing was never developed, are making big efforts to put matters right—and are focusing on the reform of nursing education as the first step. Their successes and failures may contain lessons for all of us.

The dissolution of the Soviet Union and the emergence of new nation states has brought the total of member states in the European Region to 50, including all the republics of the former USSR. It is remarkable to reflect on how recently many of the changes have occurred: few people could have predicted, at the beginning of 1989, the rapid crumbling of former Communist regimes in central and eastern Europe and the break-up of the USSR. The destruction of the Berlin wall, with all its symbolic significance, is now closely linked, politically and economically, with the hesitant moves of the 12 European Community countries towards greater unity. All this means new alliances, new conflicts, and a new European order: it brings openness to change and experiment, but it also brings disaster, most tragically in the Balkans.

Nursing, of course, is not immune to these changes. The social, economic, and political changes in every country influence health, health care, and the practice of nursing, while nurses as citizens are influenced by their environment. New health needs are emerging in Europe, not least from the consequences of war. Infectious diseases, malnutrition, high maternal and child mortality, and physical and psychological trauma are just a few of the problems now ravaging our populations—problems we are more used to seeing in other parts of the globe. In addition, health needs which were always present but were denied by the old regimes are now being openly expressed.

Countries trying to meet these old and new needs are short of money and up-to-date knowledge and skills. Reform of the health care system is high on the agenda, driven by poor standards of care, financial crisis, consumer dissatisfaction, dislike of centrally controlled structures, and ideological motives. These countries face the challenge of creating new systems which can meet demands more effectively at a time when the necessary human and financial resources are in short supply, and when the transition from command economies to mixed or market-based ones has reached a stage where neither the old nor the new systems are working.

In this environment nurses are facing many new problems, but many of the underlying difficulties are surprisingly similar to those experienced by nurses everywhere, though of course there are differences of degree. These universal themes can be summarized as power, gender and medicalization; although they exist everywhere in Europe, the issues are more acute in the former Communist countries.

Nowhere do nurses play a full part in policy-making and decision-making; many countries have no nurse in a senior ministry position and the person in charge of nursing affairs is often a physician. This lack of power is inextricably linked with the question of gender. Women make up the vast majority of the nursing workforce; men rarely number more than 10%. Nursing everywhere is women's work, and shares the characteristics of other female-dominated occupations: low pay, low status, lack of recognition, poor working conditions, few promotion prospects, and poor education. Most nurses are obliged to work what has been called the "double shift," coming home from a hard day in the hospital or community to spend their so-called spare time in caring for children, partners, and elderly or disabled family members. In caring constantly for the needs of others, nurses often find that no one is caring for them. This is particularly stressful in countries where they must spend many hours obtaining basic essentials for their families. Simply keeping the family fed and clothed is a full-time job, yet most men still regard domestic work and child care as a job for women.

Furthermore, every health system in Eastern Europe is dominated by medicine. The lion's share of prestige and resources goes to acute medical treatment, and health ministers, civil servants, and senior health service managers are nearly always doctors (usually men). Nurses are seen only as medical assistants whose job is to carry out medical orders; the caring component of healing is invisible and undervalued. The poor quality of nursing education reflects this low status. In the Soviet system, and in countries heavily influenced by it, nursing students usually started training at the age of 14 or 15. They had lectures from doctors on medical topics while continuing their general education. They had no nursing textbooks and few medical ones. Anyone who achieved high marks in their final examinations (including women) would go on to train as a doctor; nursing was only a subordinate branch of medicine.

This brief description serves to illustrate the huge scale of the task facing nursing leaders in Central and Eastern Europe and the former USSR. Although many of those practices persist, major efforts are being made to change them. Alongside heroic efforts to introduce better basic education programs in line with Council of Europe and European Community standards and directives, nurses in these countries also are working to develop specialist courses in key areas such as maternal and child health, primary health care, and psychiatry. The leaders' persistence and commitment is impressive, as is their grasp of the direction they want to follow; they are determined to shape their future by being part of the international nursing community.

They are also making good use of the policies and guidelines drawn up at the First WHO European Conference on Nursing held in Vienna in 1988. The "new role" of the European nurse is to help individuals, families, and groups to determine and achieve their physical, mental, and social potential, and to do so in the context of the environment in which they live and work. The nurse's chief functions should, therefore, be the promotion and maintenance of health, the prevention of ill health, and giving care during illness and rehabilitation. This requires the nurse to provide and manage direct nursing care; to teach patients and clients; to teach other health workers; to participate fully in the health care team; and to develop nursing practice based on critical thinking and research. More specifically, the conference made the recommendation that all basic nursing education programs be restructured, reoriented, and strengthened. This would produce generalist nurses able to function in both hospital and community and all specialist knowledge and skills could be built on this foundation.

In Eastern Europe this apparently straightforward recommendation raises interesting questions when it comes to implementation. Does it imply, for example, that basic/first-level training programs to prepare psychiatric nurses, pediatric nurses, or midwives should be phased out, and that these and similar courses should be subsumed in one broad-based common foundation program? The issue of when and how to specialize in nursing is already emerging as a dilemma in these countries. When resources are so short, is it preferable to focus first on improving basic programs, leaving specialist development for a later stage? On the other hand, if a country has acute and widely recognized needs in a specific area, such as birth control or mental health, should the priority be short-term in-service training on these topics?

Sometimes, as the WHO advisor, I am asked to lay down the law on this and other issues. WHO policies, guidelines and their underlying principles are always my starting point (Salvage, 1993), but beyond that the choice must be guided by local circumstances, and by an assessment of the real impact of each option. Only the country itself can make that choice; it is not appropriate for the WHO Regional Advisor to dictate that education courses must be 4600 hours long, or that every nurse teacher must have a degree. There is no proof that such measures would have the desired impact on health, even if they could be implemented. The imposition of a strict blueprint for nursing is neither feasible nor desirable; each country must find the solution most appropriate to its own needs and its own resources. WHO's position statements on nursing, produced by a wide cross-section of international nursing experts, are a consensus intended to provide guidance and ideas, but not instruction. In any case the top-down, imperialistic style of development work is not effective in the long term. The important, sustainable changes will be those developed and owned by the people themselves.

Whatever choices they make, nurses in every eastern European country are asking for help with the same topics—curriculum development, teacher training, and textbooks, to name only three. WHO and other international organizations can play an important role in helping colleagues to avoid duplication of effort by using our existing frameworks and guidelines, which each country, health service, or nursing school can adapt as they wish. Experience gathered from many people and situations can also help countries to minimize the problems and find good solutions and effective models of good practice.

How are colleagues in these countries coping with the challenge? At a time of such social and political turmoil, it would be surprising not to find conflict. The successful management of intraprofessional disagreement is always difficult, and all the more so in countries where the disputes between nurses mirror social, political, and cultural divisions which have become explicit since the fall of the old regimes. Dissent was formerly severely punished, and true feelings and ideas often had to be concealed, so the outburst of free expression is bound to lead to fierce argument. Using democratic group processes which respect all views and build consensus through expression of genuine differences is a new skill for most nurses, but especially for those from authoritarian regimes.

These forces, in combination with the issues of power, gender and medicalization already mentioned, add up to a daunting challenge. Yet despite the tremendous difficulties nurses face, I am constantly astonished and delighted by the energy and enthusiasm of the nurses I meet in my work. In central and eastern Europe in particular, their determination to overcome the most trying circumstances and to provide better nursing for their populations is impressive and touching. What unites nurses across Europe, and indeed across the globe, is stronger than what divides us. Events such as the Bolzano conference, where nurses come together to share knowledge and beliefs on how to improve health care, are an important way of exploring our differences but also of refreshing our altruism and our communion with fellow nurses. We have common concerns, and the best way to work on them is to look for solutions together.

REFERENCES

Salvage, J. (Ed.). (1993). *Nursing in Action: Strengthening nursing and midwifery to support health for all* (WHO Regional Publications, European Series No. 48. Copenhagen: WHO.

World Bank. (1993). *World Development Report 1993: Investing in health*. Oxford: Oxford University Press.

World Health Organization. (1989). *European conference on nursing*. Copenhagen: WHO Regional Office for Europe.

World Health Organization. (1993a). *Draft report of WHO study group on nursing beyond the year 2000*. Geneva: WHO.

World Health Organization. (1993b). *Global Advisory Group on Nursing and Midwifery: Report of the first meeting*. Geneva: WHO.

CHAPTER 2

Patterns and Samples of Nursing Education Programs Worldwide

Doris M. Modly, RN, PhD, and Ursula Springer, PhD

M any global trends in nursing education have been reviewed in Chapter 1. This chapter will discuss, in general, some of the basic patterns for nursing education found around the world. Then it will describe specific nursing education programs in nine countries from different regions of the world, to give some concrete examples of the many variations and similarities that exist among nursing education programs worldwide.

SOME BASIC PATTERNS OF NURSING EDUCATION

Nursing education is closely related to the work that nurses are expected to perform within a particular health care system. To properly understand the education programs for nurses, one must know the context in which they function. Among national health care systems there are many common features but also significant differences. All national systems of nursing education train nurses in basic elements of patient care. Generally, in countries with less developed economic and technical institutions most nurses begin their training with less education and receive shorter programs of nursing education. Countries with more advanced economic and social conditions tend to require more advanced levels of nursing education. More advanced countries also have more avenues for specialized education beyond the basic level.

Advancing the education of nurses can take several forms: at the basic level, it means requiring higher levels of schooling for entrance and giving a more substantive educational foundation. At the more advanced levels it means training more extensively in special skills, research, high technology procedures, and teaching competence.

The most basic level of nursing education provides students after completing required years of primary school education with training opportunities at hospitals. Similar to apprentices in other crafts, these nursing students learn "on the job." In some so-called developing countries this pattern may be the norm. This level is somewhat equivalent to licensed practical nurses or vocational nurses in the United States.

Countries with stronger financial resources nowadays tend to raise the entry-level of nursing students to that of 10 or 12 years of schooling, which corresponds to the high school diploma level in the United States (but not to university access in most countries). Students at this entry level usually attend nursing school for one or two years, receiving both practical and academic training. The more ambitious graduates of these nursing schools may become teachers or go on to more advanced studies. However, since nursing doctoral programs are so few, most study in related disciplines, like education, psychology, sociology, or biology.

Another advanced pattern of nursing education is obtained at the university-equivalent, but independent, higher institute, comparable to professional schools of other fields like architecture, art, engineering, etc. These higher institutes, in most countries of the world, develop outside the traditional (and generally conservative) universities. Yet the professors and students have the same official status as those of the traditional universities. Until 5 or 6 years ago, few countries saw the development of such nursing education, but since the late 1980s, small experimental programs of this type have begun. And by 1993 several countries passed legislation to raise the broad level of nursing education to required university status. In Australia, Korea, Italy, and Great Britain, the education of registered nurses had been determined to be equivalent to university studies, with the same entrance requirements. In Germany, eight Fachhochschulen (higher institutes) for nursing education were founded in 1994.

Figure 2.1 is a schematic diagram displaying a rough approximation of available nursing education options around the globe. Programs vary widely from country to country, as is made obvious later on in this chapter, when examples from specific countries are discussed.

The trend toward advancing nursing education is a great victory for nurses, who for a hundred years have labored under modest, harsh and often demeaning conditions. However, rarely does a victory come without problems. The major problem is finances. For the students, the longer studies mean foregone earnings, thus making it harder for young people from modest backgrounds to embark on longer nursing studies. For the hospitals employing the nurses with more advanced training, the salaries may be difficult to afford. The government that pays for the extended higher education for nurses must raise more taxes or higher reimbursements of general health insurance costs.

Another problem concerns career selection. In countries where all university studies are nearly free or low-cost, young people may choose medicine over nursing, if the training is not significantly longer; although the entrance requirements may be more demanding. Finally, nurses with specialized train-

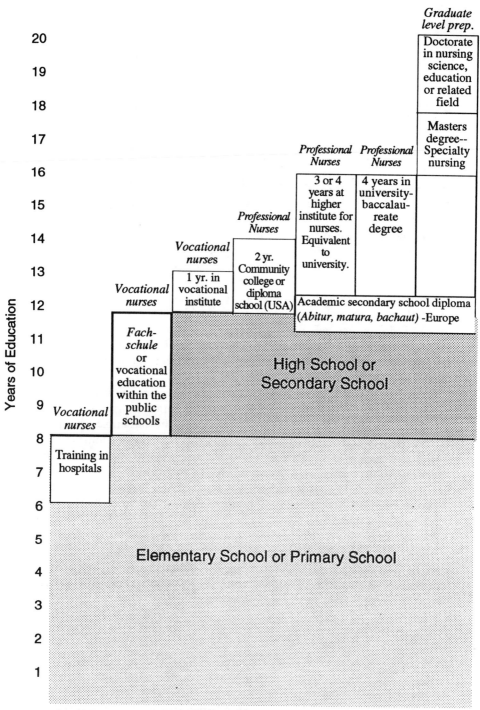

FIGURE 2.1 Various patterns of nursing education worldwide.

ing may work independently as many nurse practitioners do in the United States, where there is a shortage of physicians in primary care, and in rural areas. But in countries like Germany, Holland and other West European nations, where all university studies have been free for the past several decades, there is an oversupply of physicians and thus a disinclination to welcome competition by nurse practitioners.

A SAMPLING OF NURSING EDUCATION PROGRAMS WORLDWIDE

Nursing education worldwide occurs on several educational levels with different prerequisites for entry into the programs. Curricula in these programs prepare basically two different types of nurses for beginning practice: the "vocational" nurse, and the "registered" nurse. It must be understood, however, that several educational programs for entry into nursing practice exist simultaneously in most countries of the world. One of the major issues for the profession in general and in particular for countries that are undergoing major reform in nursing education is which of the multiple programs to eliminate while introducing new programs and still continue to meet minimal nursing care needs of the population.

A brief overview is given here of nursing education programs preparing "registered" nurses. Examples of the nursing education programs in 9 countries from different regions of the world are given. These examples should not be compared as equal units, since the educational systems of countries in the world vary a great deal. This is particularly the case in higher education, where traditions can be very strong relative to the inclusion or exclusion of persons with varied educational backgrounds.

Advanced, post-basic nursing education in most countries of the world progresses on a horizontal level. A nurse thus can be certified in several specialties of advanced practice, however, often they do not receive academic recognition. The trend globally now is to rectify this by designing vertical pathways of nursing education and moving the basic educational programs to levels of higher education and into the university. This will provide opportunities for upward mobility in the academic world.

Hungary

In Hungary, as in all countries of Central Europe, nursing education is in a process of fundamental restructuring. Until recently, most students of nursing began their nursing education on the secondary school level. Upon completion of basic nursing education, that lasted 3 or 4 years, graduates were certified as beginning nurses who within a year had to complete a first level advanced preparation in one nursing specialty to be permitted continued practice as nurses. These educational programs will be phased out by 1996. Since the majority of nurses practicing currently in Hungary have the above described basic education, opportunities will be provided for them to bridge into a new program if they so desire and academically qualify.

Under the mandates of the restructuring, all those entering basic schools of nursing beginning with 1996, must have completed secondary school or 12 years of general education, including the successful completion of the educational "competency" exam. Two types of programs are even now open to those students: 3-year programs that are not university based and 4-year, higher education/university based programs. Both types meet the requirements of the European Union: the minimum age of entry is 16 years, the program is 4600 hours in length, with a minimum of at least one half of the hours to be clinical learning situations. Required courses and their minimum course content is prescribed. The 4-year program is based in a college of health sciences. Entry into the program requires a university level entrance examination. Minimum nursing requirements are the same as in the three-year program, however, additional liberal education is included in the curriculum.

Nicaragua

In Nicaragua a professional nursing education, called "basico," consists of a 3-year course of study following the completion of secondary school or 12 years of general education. Auxiliary nurses may begin training after nine years of general education requirements are met. Specialty training consists of a short course to augment skills but without postgraduate credit.

Egypt

Egypt also provides nursing education on secondary school levels, both in secondary grammar schools and vocational schools. These programs prepare nurse generalists as well as specialists, such as midwives and maternal–child health nurses. Recently, university affiliated Higher Institutes of Nursing have been established at several universities in Egypt. Advanced learning programs at the masters level as well as the doctoral level also exist.

Ireland

Nursing in Ireland commands a high degree of respect; thus, Ireland experiences more applications to nursing programs than there are slots in schools. These programs are under statutory control and comply with the European Union's requirements for general nursing. The educational system consists of basic, pre-registration, and post-basic education programs. Pre-registration education is mainly an apprenticeship education, positioned under the Department of Health. Academic points are not given for the study of basic nursing.

Nurses in Ireland have been working to introduce changes. A university based, three year, basic nursing program was opened at University College Galway leading to a college diploma. In post-basic education, nurse tutors can obtain a nursing baccalaureate degree at University College, Department of Nursing Studies in Dublin, where a basic education program is being developed in affiliation with the College of Surgeons. Non-degree, post-basic studies in different specialty areas can be completed in 6 months to 1 year.

USA

In the United States, most nursing education occurs at the community college level with transfers to baccalaureate programs made possible with relative ease. Hospital-based diploma schools still exist, but are diminishing in number. For many years they were the most prevalent form of nursing education. In recent years, educational opportunities have been developed for hospital-based, diploma school graduates to obtain a baccalaureate degree in nursing, because the trend for baccalaureate and masters level of education has become a requirement for advanced practice and certification in many nursing specialties and for nurse practitioner certification. Recently, an increasing number of non-nurse college graduates are choosing nursing as a professional career and enrolling in clinical masters and doctorate programs that prepare them for basic and advanced practice in nursing.

Canada

In Canada most nurses are educated at the diploma level in community colleges. A few remaining hospital schools are affiliated with community colleges that provide the non-nursing courses. A small percentage of nurses obtain their basic nursing education in 4-year, university degree programs. Degree-prepared nurses provide basic nursing care in communities, as managers and as clinical teachers.

Australia

After a review of nursing education in Australia was carried out during the early 1980s, the government of Australia transferred all hospital-based nursing education to the higher education sector. The transfer was carried out gradually in order to lessen the disruption to the health care system. All nursing education is now government supported. Entry into nursing programs requires completion of year 12 of a secondary school program. There are two types of 3-year basic nursing education programs, one leading to the BSc degree in nursing and a 3-year college program that leads to a Diploma in Nursing. Post-basic nursing courses prepare specialists in the different clinical specialties.

Thailand

Currently, there are two entry level nursing education programs offered in Thailand: the four-year baccalaureate program and the two-year technical nurse program. Students are selected by nationwide or institutional entrance examinations following twelve years of general schooling, or high school graduation. Upon successful completion of the four-year university-level nursing program, students are prepared for entry level practice in nursing. They are awarded the baccalaureate degree in nursing science and are admissible for graduate study on the masters and doctoral level. The two-year technical program prepares students for the practice of nursing as technical nurses. This group represents the majority of nurses currently in practice. A 2-year college level program aims to assist technical nurses who have been in nursing practice at least 2 years to upgrade themselves. The baccalaureate degree is awarded after 2 years of study, making graduates of this program eligible for graduate study at a university.

The diploma in nursing programs prepared entry level nurses in the past. These programs are now closed. Diploma prepared registered nurses, however, continue in practice. A 1-year B.S.N. program aims to develop their competencies and prepare them for graduate study in nursing.

Zimbabwe

Not unlike many countries of the world, nursing education in Zimbabwe is in flux. The aim of all change in Zimbabwe is to upgrade nursing education to prepare nurses for the responsibilities they face in a country that does not have enough health care providers, particularly physicians.

In Zimbabwe at the present time, basic nursing education also occurs on several educational levels. These different nursing education programs have different requisites for entry and they lead to different levels of competence upon completion. Programs leading to state certification, the designation "State Certified Nurse" (S.C.N.), is based on completed secondary education with three "O" level exams. The length of the program is 2 years. This program is now discontinued and SCN nurses still in the system have an opportunity to participate in a 1-year program to qualify as State Registered Nurses. Students preparing to become State Registered Nurses are those who enter a three year program having completed five "O" level and two or more "A" level exams. This group represents the majority of nurses in Zimbabwe. Most practicing nurses, however, have advanced education in a specialty, but without academic recognition. A basic Baccalaureate program in nursing has been approved and will be implemented in the near future.

TABLE 2.1 Programs of Nursing Education for "Certified & Registered" Nurses

Level of Education Required to Enter/Program Level	Length of Program	Acad. degree (title) received	License	Country
Secondary school level without certificate of maturity*	3 years	-	Nursing Certificate	Hungary Nicaragua
Secondary school level with certificate of maturity	4 years	High school Diploma	Nursing Certificate	Hungary Egypt
Post secondary school level/hospital based	3 years	Nursing Diploma	Registered Nurse	Ireland
Post secondary school level/based in schools of nursing	3 years	-	Registered Nurse	Hungary Nicaragua USA
Post secondary school/higher education level	2 years	AD/degree	Registered Nurse	USA Canada Thailand Australia
Post secondary school/higher education level	3 years 4 years	Diploma of Higher Education	Registered Nurse	Australia Hungary Ireland
Post secondary school/university level	4 years	BSN Degree	Registered Nurse	Thailand USA Egypt
Post undergraduate/graduate level	4 years	ND Degree	Registered Nurse/Adv. Practice	USA
Post secondary school and 3 O exam level**	2 years	-	State Certified Nurse	Zimbabwe
Post secondary school and 5 O exam level 2 A exam level***	3 years	-	State Certified Nurse	Zimbabwe

*Certificate of maturity = completion of study & successful passing of a comprehensive exam, which is a requirement for university admission (primarily in Europe)
**O level exams are = ordinary level exam required for completion of secondary school (British system)
***A level exams are = advanced level exams, taken after passing O level exams, allows for university admission (British system)

CHAPTER 3

Broadening Nursing Boundaries Through Nursing Education and Nursing Education Research

Renzo Zanotti, IP, AFD, PhD

CULTURE AND BOUNDARIES

In this last decade of the century, we are witness to the extraordinary evolution of human society. Amazing social paradoxes and dramatic changes in the map of the world are challenging our capacity to deal with the emerging diversity. Old behaviors are still in effect, and war, fear, and pain are still present. Social and professional scenarios are more complex, exciting, and contradictory than a decade ago. Some traditional walls have fallen, but they have been quickly replaced with new ones. The human being seems to be unable to cope with the diversity and accept the difference as a resource. Personal needs of certainty and safety and different forms of educational stigmata are boundaries continually present, driving our perception and construction of reality. As part of our thought, these boundaries between our subjectivity and "reality" follow us in our private life, at school, on the job, and everywhere. Therefore, boundaries are always present within ourselves because they are settled in our cultural imprinting, in our mental constructs, in our personal epistemology of the world. We are living expressions of our boundaries, with our behaviors, our cultural patterns, our tireless judging of the world (and other human beings), too, often assuming that our mental, subjective, symbolized reality is the paramount reality.

Boundaries are delimitations; a boundary certifies a difference between what is on one side and what is on the other; they are used to separate contents within professional and disciplinary domains when they deal with similar phenomena. The necessity of boundaries among allied disciplines is advocated by the members in order to clarify their differences and uniqueness. Separation through delineation of a boundary sometimes produces an amplification of that difference, and this can result in more gratification for the members of specific domains. As a consequence, the boundaries are used sometimes just for keeping disciplines strong and underlining differences; otherwise, these disappear. Boundaries are often used as cultural definitions of hypothetical entities, as symbols, as labels.

23

NURSING: A HUMAN CULTURE FOR THE HUMAN BEING

Within the nature of a human being there is a tendency to separate, and a tendency to come nearer. Both are present in the social human behaviors and cultural expressions of human beings.

Nursing is historically an expression of human mercy, traditionally more connotating attitudes, passion, and dedication, than is science. Nursing has always been represented by the bedside nurse, with a closer relationship to the patient than any other health professional. The nurse prototype is "able to feel" the patient's needs and respond "person-to-person" with a unique expression of humanity, dedication, and professional attitude. Despite the triumph of positivism in Western culture in the last century, nursing knowledge remained different, pushed by the professional, technical, and social evolution toward a strong competition with the allied disciplines in order to achieve a higher scientific prestige, but, at the same time, remaining tied to its roots in humanistic culture.

The question of competition is now, more than ever, an important topic in the health field. Competition, first of all, to achieve a higher social rank and scientific prestige; but also a better professional practice and unique cultural identity. Competition among allied disciplines is a sign of their overlapping domains but it is also motivational energy, challenging thinkers and theorists to look for new elements of uniqueness, and scientists to provide evidence using research methods supporting the value of theoretical statements in explaining and predicting aspects of the reality.

Differentiation is a natural process of human social development: differentiation is the distinctive feature of a complex culture. Cultural differentiation is also a troublesome concept in nursing, eternally trying to express its originality in regard to the allied disciplines and at the same time originating new professions from itself. As the body of nursing culture grows, new subfields emerge, fueling the debate, internally on nursing's social mandate and domain. Both dimensions internal and external to nursing are in many ways narrowly embedded. First, because the knowledge implemented in nursing education is largely based on biology, psychology, sociology, education, medicine, and other disciplines. Second, because the nursing clinical areas of knowledge came from, in content and label, the original medical culture. The medical model can often be found behind the modern concept of nursing specialization. The growing tendency in many countries to split professional knowledge into specialized clinical sectors can be questioned, if these sectors are founded mostly on medical specialties or if, in some ways, the nursing specialties follow the medical example; because one consequence is that the specialized nurse becomes a "clinical specialist," usually more adept at managing events and decisions from a medical perspective within a very narrow field, than managing people, diversity, and change. On the other hand, starting in some countries from a different ideology, the unique figure of the nurse is proposed as an alternative to professional fragmentation and cultural specialization. This "all in one" nurse should be trained more in processes and problem-solving during academic preparation; that means a need for continuing education in different clinical settings during professional activity. This program envisions a nurse as a "complete professional," with little concern for technical sophisticated expertise. These two perspectives, specialization and integration, are expressions of different philosophies and social expectations.

Behind the nursing programs there are cultural models, philosophical assumptions, and social needs. As a consequence, nursing education is largely shaped by the country's culture, social model, and health system. However, despite the influence of national issues on professional education, basic nursing ideals are rooted in the cross-cultural values of human solidarity and a person's uniqueness, and a common dedication to the professional practice of caring. Common ideals and values and different backgrounds, training and social mandates are ingredients that characterize nursing across national boundaries. Strongly acknowledged worldwide for a humanitarian attitude, the nurse still lacks a clear scientific identity acknowledged by society. In fact, after decades of debate, the uniqueness of nursing as a disciplinary field, so strongly perceived and advocated by nurses, is not yet a closed question. Moreover, the movement from a practice profession to a professional discipline is a slow process that proceeds with different speed within the different areas and settings of nursing. Academic nursing and practice are often split. On the academic side, there are philosophical speculations, conceptual developments, and theory testing that feed the body of knowledge and enlarge the disciplinary dimension. However, this is mostly concentrated in a few countries, where by history, resources, and social mandate nursing research can receive appropriate economic and organizational resources. As a consequence, nursing disciplinary culture is produced mostly by countries considered dominant and is often rejected by other countries. On the other side, there is the practice, where organizational rules, economic concerns, and medically oriented education propel the priority of the tasks. In contrast to the disciplinary culture, where the human being is the focus, there is a "practice theory" based on the local hospital culture that drives the activities of caring and shapes its values.

Nursing is a complex idea and has a complex, heterogeneous educational system. The disparate ways, across nations, of teaching nursing are often neither known, nor compared, nor recognized for their potential contribution, nor appreciated. Dealing with our cultural diversities and struggling with our common basic questions can allow us to think, to learn, to teach the culture of nursing as a common pattern, beyond the frontiers, beyond our uncertainty, targeting the human being's health as a unifying phenomena.

The modern fast-developing health sciences are a powerful aggregate force relating to common phenomena of the health care field, despite national and cultural differences. Intensifying ethnic differences and increasing science integration seem to be the main paradox of this decade. With this apparent contradiction, nursing could be a disciplinary expression of a unified culture, bridging science and humanism, still able to understand the person's health needs and struggling to satisfy them, regardless of all the cultural and ethnic differences.

THE CHALLENGE IS TO BROADEN NURSING EDUCATION BY INCORPORATING A MULTICULTURAL PERSPECTIVE

The first goal for nursing as a discipline beyond nationality for the health of human beings, is the implementation of a multicultural perspective in professional programs. Educating with a multicultural perspective is consistent with the basic disciplinary value that the health of the person is the paramount phenomenon of interest, regardless of race, culture, sex, and religion. Education for nursing should be not merely an acquisition of some professional skills but, above all, the acquisition of a distinctive epistemology in which scientific knowledge is driven by ethical values and humanistic philosophy.

Teaching nursing requires that educators be aware that the disciplinary focus is on the fascinating complexity of the health of the human being. Understanding this complexity without reducing the whole to its parts is the real cultural goal of nursing education. Holism, person as a system, person as a whole, should not be merely slogans or traditional values for nursing culture but a real expression of nurses' philosophy; the framework driving the practice. Education to nursing should not be just a question of teaching contents and teaching methods, but primarily an awareness of cultural identity and disciplinary epistemology. Education is the key, the first tool for preparing a person to be an active member, a real resource for human society and the discipline: we need to educate future nurses to listen, to talk, to compare without prejudice, to learn from each other, and to develop skills to cope with uncertainty.

THE SECOND CHALLENGE: ENHANCE NURSING EDUCATION WORLDWIDE THROUGH NURSING EDUCATION RESEARCH

Research is the only way to produce scientific knowledge. Systematic knowledge is a most unifying product for the disciplinary culture. Sharing a common vision of nursing's uniqueness requires us jointly to update our culture and share research findings. We need educators and researchers who are able to produce and diffuse knowledge valid for different cultures using cross-cultural tools and concepts. Research could be an heuristic way to educate toward new forms of thought, where discovery and rational thought are joined together.

Many peculiarities across countries are uncharted and research is needed to better evaluate possible relationships between nursing models that are working and the environment that originated them. These national, still isolated, experiences and educational experiments must find an organized structure that allows their systematic comparison, description, and report for periodical analysis of the disciplinary state of the art.

Enhancing the contribution of scientific knowledge in the body of disciplinary culture permits also to reduce the influence of national cultures and particular components on nursing's disciplinary perspective, and will facilitate a common definition of strategies, instruments, and procedures worldwide. More scientific knowledge requires better training in research for students, instructors, and professors in a pervasive model that starts at the entry-level schools. Since the long tradition of nursing as art and practical profession, many generations of nurses have not been prepared either to use scientifically based criteria in their decisions, or to perceive the profession as research-based. Many nurses are not educated to perceive themselves as an active part of the research process; for example, raising questions, defining problems, communicating cases and events, and applying research findings into practice. The contribution of the individual nurse could be invaluable for nursing science. They should be considered for advanced education programs with a specific concern for enlarging their skills, in order to be more adept in sharing the advances in the profession, reading scientific literature, and facing new challenges as a part of a scientific and professional community.

Facilitating multisite research, supporting a wider use of the scientific literature in entry-level nursing programs, exchanging nursing faculty internationally, and improving the frequency and quality of international meetings can produce a significant feature of nursing's uniqueness: its international culture, beyond all the frontiers and cultural rigidity of this troubled world.

CHAPTER 4

Trends in U.S. Health Services: Implications for Practice and Education

Mary O. Mundinger, RN, PhD, FAAN

N ursing practice is changing globally, and with these changes, nursing education must build a new infrastructure. In the United States these changes mean that nurses will have more autonomy and authority, especially advanced practice nurses (APNS). This is true both for primary care practice and for hospitals, where APNs will increasingly take on the full responsibility and care of critically ill but stable patients. Those who are medically unstable and in need of complex medical diagnoses and care will remain under the primary authority of physicians, but nurses will have authority for others.

APNs must have similar education and competencies worldwide if we expect acceptance and agreement on their role. Until now, nursing competence has been similar according to educational background, but legal, professional, and financial barriers have limited scope of practice. Nursing must make a concerted effort to base scope of practice on education and competency, not on local limitations that are more often based on anticompetitive concerns rather than on competency. The best example of this in the United States is the Medicare statute, which gives nurse practitioners full authority and full reimbursement in rural areas where there is a shortage of physicians, but not in areas where there are sufficient numbers of physicians.

Universal standards will allow and promote international exchange of scholars. With common expectations for APN practice, interchanges will be facilitated. There are four imperatives for the profession. First is differentiated practice, which means that scope of practice is determined by educational achievements. In the United States today we do not differentiate hospital nursing roles by educational degrees, and this confuses the public about what different degrees authorize nurses to do. We must be clear that advanced practice always requires a Master's degree and that community nursing requires a Baccalaureate degree. The second imperative is universal standards for APNs. Advance practice nursing not only requires a Master's degree, but the content of that training should be similar across geographical boundaries. Similar competencies should also be outlined and adhered to.

Third, we must set new research priorities. Nursing research historically has been focused on educational issues, on nursing theory development or testing, and more recently, on nursing practice. In the future we must claim our place as evaluators of patient health outcomes, treatment effectiveness, cost effectiveness, and technology assessment (what works in what setting for identified health problems). When nursing was a young science, and when most care was not determined and ordered by nurses, the more traditional research priorities were sufficient; that is no longer the case. As nursing's authority grows, so must the scope of its research.

Finally, there will be new partnerships with medicine and with nursing teams. Medicine and nursing will form teams of equal partners, with equal authority for different aspects of care, and with growing areas of overlapping competency. These overlap areas will increasingly go to nursing, because nurses handle them more cost-effectively and because medical knowledge is growing as fast as nursing, making it imperative that nurses provide the more basic care previously provided only by physicians. New nursing teams also will be formed. APNs will take on more authoritative roles in hospital care and will be determining the care that other nurses give. It may indeed be more difficult to distinguish these new nurse-to-nurse relationships than the new relationships between physicians and nurses.

The paraprofessional work force also will grow. As the United States population becomes more ethnically diverse, and as we acknowledge that effective care requires attention to cultural values and lifestyles, it will become imperative to include caregivers who reflect the cultures and lifestyles of our patients. Our professional training programs will increasingly include cultural and ethnic minorities, and the paraprofessional work force can include minorities, and particularly immigrants, very quickly.

IMPENDING CHANGES IN THE HEALTH CARE SYSTEM

Dynamics among professionals will change. APNs and physicians will craft new, more integrative roles. The structure of care and reimbursement will also change. Care will less likely be covered as episodic periods, and more often will be configured as a seamless continuum for every consumer, so that health promotion and disease prevention activities will be ongoing even when illness is not being treated. Reimbursement more often will be capitated, with providers receiving an annual fee for which the consumer will receive all needed care. This system may be refined to pay more for better outcomes, rather than the current system, which pays more for more care without assessing the outcome. Perhaps one day we will adopt the Chinese system, which pays the doctor when his patient stays well and provides sickness care free.

Other changes will affect research priorities, practice opportunities, the site of care, and partnerships for inpatient management. Outcome and effectiveness research will take precedence. The greater emphasis on primary care will mean that most care will be provided in community settings, rather than in institutions, and that there will be more community sites for disease prevention and health promotion. There will be more cross-site care, where the same provider will follow his/her patient across sites from community to hospital to home. Physicians and nurses will share authority for inpatient management.

Differentiated practice will be a main concern of future health policy. Without clear indicators of what educational level signifies what level of practice, policymakers will limit practice to the lowest common denominator. At this time, nursing makes no distinctions among the Baccalaureate-prepared nurse, the diploma-prepared nurse, or the nurse with an associate's degree for bedside nursing. In fact, in most situations it is difficult to demonstrate that the Baccalaureate prepared nurse practices differently in the hospital situation from the licensed practical nurse. Policymakers, in order to assure and guarantee patient safety, can only allow nurses to practice at the minimum level of practice that everyone is able to provide. If we cannot show that different educational preparation leads to different functions, then policy can allow only the level of practice that every nurse in that role performs. It behooves us in the profession to begin setting guidelines for practice that are different for different levels of education. In this way policy can allow higher levels of authority for those with higher levels of education.

Nurse educators must do more with colleagues in service to make these distinctions clear. Without a clear consensus between leaders in nursing education and service, we will not be able to provide the appropriate education as the infrastructure for the differentiated practice levels.

Nursing also must carry out research to show how formal learning correlates with practice competency. In order to lend credibility to differentiated practice, and differentiated education as the basis for differentiated practice, we need research to show us how education leads to levels of practice competency. Do Baccalaureate-prepared nurses practice differently? Do they achieve different outcomes?

Nursing needs to articulate the different levels of nursing practice within which a nurse can learn and develop from novice to expert. Part of the reason we have been reluctant to differentiate practice is because we are uncomfortable saying that Baccalaureate level education is better, or of higher quality, or provides more expertise than Associate Degree education. We should, rather, be clarifying that becoming an expert has to do with practicing at the greatest competency within the goals and expectations of a specific educational background. Therefore the Associate Degree-prepared nurse becomes an expert by doing at a very high skill level, and the Baccalaureate-prepared nurse becomes an expert by planning at a high skill level. This is a somewhat simplistic explanation, since we know baccalaureate prepared nurses give direct care expertly and that Associate Degree-prepared nurses are called upon to plan care as well as give it, but expertise for the two educational backgrounds is different. If we can say that each level has distinct areas of expertise and value, but that the practice differs, we are more likely to have policy which permits a higher level of practice authority for those who are clearly prepared for it.

A second concern of health policy will be establishing international standards for advanced practice, in terms of curricula, practice scope, and certification. The time has come for the international nursing community to agree on basic curricula for different levels of practice. What is needed for the care of acutely ill, institutionalized patients? What is needed for public health, community-based, and home care practice? What is needed for the preparation of nurses in primary care?

As concerns practice scope, while technology and relationships with physicians differ internationally—and indeed differ even between urban and rural—there are a number of commonalities that the international community can agree on. These are diagnostic scope, treatment protocols, and practice guidelines that both physicians and nurses can use.

Common standards and criteria for certification can begin to be developed internationally as the curricula and practice scope are agreed upon. We need to expand the boundaries and decrease the barriers to patient access for professional nurses everywhere.

PARTNERSHIPS AND NEW TEAMS

Nursing Teams

The following people might make up a nursing team: A Baccalaureate-prepared nurse, who will act as team leader and handle discharge planning and community care; an Associate Degree nurse who will be a bedside nurse; aides; and technicians. Technology takes up significant time and expense in the care of patients. Professional care, from those who plan and decide when and for what purpose care is given, is largely wasted in the actual repetitive giving of technological care. It can be provided more cost-effectively by technicians.

The advanced practice nurse in acute care is a clinical specialist and is moving into more direct care for medically complex patients within the hospital setting. Much of this advancement in authority overlaps with what physicians have done in the past. Nurses must be sure to develop these new roles not only with physicians, but with their nursing colleagues.

Families can be involved in care cooperatively with professionals, both in the hospital and in community sites. This makes the patient more likely to adopt the care regimen and gives family members a sense of contribution to the person's healing. Many hospitals have adopted Cooperative Care Units with great success.

Culturally diverse and sensitive nurses are essential. We are entering an era when the biggest advances in health will not come from technology, but from adherence to proven helpful regimens of care, from lifestyle changes, from targeted risk assessment, and from specific measures for disease prevention and health promotion. For these modalities to be optimally helpful, we must take into consideration the cultural values of the patients being served. In the hospital, in the community, and particularly in patients' homes, care must be reflective of values and beliefs to be fully adopted. We should be doing more to empower members of our minority and culturally diverse populations in health care roles. They bring an added dimension to our efforts to have patients adopt more healthful lives.

Nursing-Medical Teams

Such teams will be newly developed outside, as well as within, the hospital.

- *Continuity Care Models with Physician Consultation*: In this model, Advanced Practice Nurses take the lead in diagnosing and treating patients across sites, from community or office into the hospital and back to their homes. Nurses admit for nursing care, and physicians are called in to provide consultation and intervention when needed.
- *First-Year Medical Residents Overlap for APN Practice*: In this model, APNs function in roles traditionally reserved for first-year medical residents. Much of what residents do serves patients, rather than adding to residents' own advanced learning. As the number of hospital residents declines and more receive their training in community sites, APNs will fill the void of inpatient service.
- *Primary Care Teams with Nursing*: In this model nurses will carry out the first contact and comprehensive diagnostic and management work, while MDs will be responsible for the more complex diagnoses and interventions.

Nursing's new roles vis-á-vis medicine must be reflected in a redesigned curriculum, both for physicians and for nurses. By changing the educational content and the multidisciplinary context in which they will practice, students are socialized differently and unnecessary curricular overlaps are eliminated.

There are a number of reasons why advanced practice nursing is good for physicians. First, physicians train too long for primary care. Education is too expensive for the resulting rewards in practice. Second, the focus and interest of physicians are incompatible with needs in primary care, which are primarily the uncomplicated detection and treatment of illness, health education, and disease prevention. Third, doctors do not know community or family resources very well, nor are they particularly interested in working to advance these resources.

Finally, specialty physicians maintain a proportion of their practice in the provision of primary care, because they value seeing patients over time; because many patients requiring specialty care also require primary care; and because they can fill out their practices with primary care at specialty prices. The problem with this is that they provide primary care through the prism of their specialty. Thus cardiologists are more likely to order a stress test and gastroenterologists a colonoscopy, regardless of the presenting history and symptoms of the patient. If physicians collaborate with nurses, there are a number of advantages. First, they will lower their liability, for a doctor/nurse team is more likely to give comprehensive user-friendly care. Secondly, they will increase the marketing of their practice because of the comprehensiveness and cost-effectiveness of team care. Third, they will escape from care that is not interesting to them by having an APN take on those aspects of practice.

In summary, educational imperatives for nursing should be:

- Develop curriculum and model new roles with physicians, with nurse colleagues, in new sites, doing new things;
- Engage in new partnerships with nursing service to develop the roles and conduct the research needed to support differentiated practice;
- Engage in new partnerships with medicine in practice and education;
- Develop research competencies in meta-analysis and technology assessment, skills that will be needed to carry on practice research in the future;
- Redefine the social contract in higher education and make sure student experiences more fully benefit patients. We know that our graduates meet the social contract, but it is not clear that we have fully developed our educational programs to assure that student practice has a productivity component;
- Form international coalitions to standardize advanced practice nursing;
- Advance nursing research internationally including multi-site development of studies to address common research questions; and
- Advance the international exchange of students and faculty.

PART II

Teaching Practices Worldwide

CHAPTER 5

Designing Curriculum to Advance Nursing Science and Professional Practice

Doris M. Modly, RN, PhD

> *Education is not acquiring a stock of ready-made ideas, images, sentiments, beliefs, and so forth; it is learning to listen, to think, to feel, to imagine, to believe, to understand, to choose and to wish.*

> (Oakeshott, 1989, pp. 66–67)

In the second half of the twentieth century, heavy emphasis has been placed on the development of nurse scholars and researchers, first in the United States (Fitzpatrick & Abraham, 1988), and more recently in other countries of the world where nursing scholarship is recognized as necessary for quality research and quality practice that is grounded in nursing knowledge.

Nursing research courses have been introduced in all baccalaureate nursing programs, to enable learners to read the research literature and to use appropriately research findings in practice. One nursing research course, however, does not suffice to meet the needs of science. What then are the characteristics of a curriculum that facilitates the development of practice competencies and at the same time fosters the potential in practitioners to advance the scientific discipline of nursing and enhance the development of nursing practice in the future? Perhaps one such characteristic is temporal orientation: i.e., whether or not the curriculum is oriented to the present or future.

The contrast between the temporal orientation of professional nursing practice, which is aimed at meeting present-day health care or nursing care needs of people, and the orientation of science, which anticipates and prepares for the practice of the future, leads to the question: What is to be the priority when a curriculum for the education of professional nurses is designed—the needs of present-day practice or the development of future practice? Since both are important, the challenge is how best to design a basic nursing curriculum that is both practice- and science-oriented.

Pressures to prepare competent "doers" of nursing invariably confront the educator with the imperative to assure that graduates know how to provide

37

appropriate nursing care for today's patients. Graduates of any nursing education program must meet the health and nursing care needs of the population they are to serve, no matter where in the world a program is implemented. This is irrefutable. As professional practitioners, however, nurses must also be prepared to create the future of their practice discipline. Therefore, the development of inquiring students requires careful consideration when a curriculum is constructed.

In this chapter factors which influence the process of curriculum construction and implementation are discussed; these factors ultimately determine the general competencies of graduates. Some of these variables are external to the program and are difficult to manipulate, such as the context in which education and practice occur. Others are internal to the educational system and can be influenced by nurse educators and by the profession in general.

MEETING EDUCATIONAL NEEDS IN THE CONTEXT OF PRACTICE

The development of the ADN (Associate in Nursing Degree) program in the United States in the early 1950s is an example of nursing education meeting the needs of the present. The United States emerged from World War II more conscious than ever of its need for highly trained nurses (Haase, 1990). The great need at the time was for more nurses with technical nursing skills. An innovative curriculum was designed that not only met that social need but also provided a means for nursing education to advance from the apprenticeship, service-based model to a knowledge-based model of higher education. When community college education became prominent, many women interested in nursing sought education in these community college programs. Repeated nursing shortages, combined with the desire of nurse leaders to remove nursing education from the control of service agencies, led to the rapid expansion of ADN programs nationwide.

Funding from both governmental and non-governmental agencies propelled this reform in nursing education, which resulted in the closing of most hospital-based schools of nursing in the USA by 1985. Thus, nursing education moved out of the service domain into the mainstream of higher education and met society's needs for nursing services in the present.

The major change in the ADN programs from the traditional curricula of diploma programs was a shift in emphasis from the patient's disease, as in the medicine oriented hospital schools of nursing, to the patient's or client's needs. With innovative methods of instruction, organization of assignments, and testing, these 2-year programs prepared students to perform the functions assigned to registered nurses and practice in the here and now. The success of these programs can be measured by the fact that more than half of all registered nurses who graduated in 1983, and 37% of all nurses registered in the USA that year, were ADN graduates (Haase, 1990). Educational upward mobility in recent years has enabled many ADN nurses to attain a baccalaureate degree in nursing (BSN).

An example designed to meet the society's needs on a local level was a basic nursing education program at the Frances Payne Bolton School of Nursing of Case Western Reserve University. After ten years of only graduate-level nursing education, a baccalaureate program was reinstituted in the early 1990s in response to the local health care community's needs for more intensive/tertiary care nurses. An opportunity for extensive clinical experience was built into the fourth year of the program in order to prepare nurses for the increasing acuity of patients in tertiary care settings and enable graduates to have a shorter orientation to the highly technical environment of intensive care units.

Through collaboration with three major tertiary care hospitals that need baccalaureate-prepared and technically skilled nurses, the school is able to offer students major support for tuition and guaranteed employment in the participating hospitals for 2 years after graduation. The objective is to educate nurses with a clinical "focus" and competency in beginning practice in acute and critical care nursing. The curriculum of this program is strongly practice-oriented. However, since the program is housed in a major research university, whose mission is the development of science, the program is also science-oriented, and it prepares students to recognize the knowledge base of their practice. Students are introduced to nursing research as well as technical advances in health care delivery, e.g., informatics and the use of computers in health care delivery. Students observe advanced practice in the clinical settings where they learn, e.g., nurse-managed intensive care units and community-based nursing clinics. The program's heavy emphasis on learning clinical practice, however, does not always guarantee students sufficient time to think creatively—a possibility that always exists when much is required within a short time.

The current emphasis on primary health care globally is requiring further changes in nursing curricula. In primary health care, nurses become involved with communities to assist them in determining their own health care. Nurses must work collaboratively with the communities toward meeting their health care needs. This direction in health care means that the role of the nurse is changing, which requires changes in curricular structure and content. The philosophy and principles of primary health care cannot be restricted to nurse practitioner curricula; rather, the basic concepts of primary health care also must be included in basic nursing education. Similarly, home-based care is requiring new directions in the education of nurses, not only in the USA, but also in most other regions of the world.

Major changes are now occurring in the educational programs for nurses in the former Soviet-bloc countries. They need to put nursing education on a par with nursing education in other European countries and to have a cadre of nurses who meet the standards for nursing practice in their own rapidly changing health care delivery systems. Most of these countries would like to model nursing education on the systems of the Western European countries in order to assure reciprocity of licenses within the Council of Europe. The practice of beginning nursing education at the conclusion of general education, that is, at the age of 14 or 15, is no longer considered desirable. Graduates of these programs are too young to shoulder the complex nursing care needs of patients; thus graduates leave nursing in large numbers shortly after completing their course of study. This in turn creates a perpetual nursing shortage, making the career even less appealing. For those who remain, continuing education and some advancement is possible, but continuing education in nursing is only on a horizontal level without access to higher education. University level education in the health care field is provided only in medicine. Nurses who desire a university education have to attain that in another discipline, and they do so most frequently in education. No academic mobility is possible in the field of nursing.

To change this requires major changes not only in nursing education but in the general education structures of these countries. All potential changes, however are highly dependent on changes in the countries' economic and welfare infrastructures. In addition to the low level of educational preparation and emotional immaturity of nurse novices, the minimum wages paid for nurses' work contributes to the undesirable image that nursing has in the eyes of the public. Thus nursing does not attract "the best and the brightest." The energy needed for a future orientation and advancement of science and professional practice is nonexistent in the curricula and there is even less opportunity for the conscious development of a nursing science based practice. The emphasis is on "doing and on assisting with" medical procedures. This fragmented, specialized care takes the attention of students and practicing nurses away from a holistic, caring attention to the needs of patients. Most very young nursing students are not able to combine knowledge, skills, and caring, particularly when the work environment does not reinforce what they hear in the classroom. Thus, in the countries of the former socialist bloc, a new need has emerged for different nursing care, which in turn mandates a change in the structure and content of basic nursing education curricula. An emphasis on humanistic, caring approaches to patients has become a mandate for change.

In most Central European countries, the aim now is to move the basic education of nurses to post-secondary school levels to assure that better educated and more mature students will study nursing. Faculty recognize that more will be required in the new curricula than just additional content to prepare practitioners for the next millennium. The new curricula will have to prepare students for practice in the here and now and at the same time equip them to create the knowledge base for future practice. Changes in this direction are underway, with a new emphasis on preparation for practice as well as the science of nursing.

Countries of other continents are facing even more rapid changes in their health care delivery systems. Nursing education must change in these countries also to meet the requirements of practice. The temptation to medicalize nursing education may be lessened because it is balanced by governments' emphasis on primary health care, in which most cases is delivered by non-physician providers. Nursing education is thus easier to move toward emphasizing health when primary health care is the focus. However, underdeveloped secondary education makes it difficult to develop the requirements of science within a curriculum.

MEETING CURRICULAR NEEDS FOR SCIENCE

The introduction of new or additional content into curricula is one way to begin to serve both the practice needs and the science of nursing. Combining the future orientation of science and the present orientation of clinical practice, however, requires more than a new curricular structure and the introduction of new courses, or new settings for instruction. A curriculum that both promotes a future orientation through the development of science and facilitates competence in the "doing" of nursing in the present, mandates a fundamental change in how nursing education is viewed and how the curriculum is implemented by teachers. If educators only change the environment in which students study and add a few new subjects, but do not change their own philosophy of nursing and of teaching and learning, changes in the thinking and practice of graduates cannot be expected.

THE DIFFERENCE BETWEEN TRAINING AND EDUCATION

A curriculum designed for practice in the present and the development of the science upon which future practice will rest must engage teachers who educate rather than those who only train. Teachers must first understand the difference between "training" and "education" (Bevis, 1988) and know when to train and how to educate. One difference between training and education lies in the relationship of the teacher and the student. In education the teacher is a facilitator of learning; in training the teacher simply conveys knowledge. An educator fosters students' independent learning and supports their creativity and critical thinking while adhering to high standards of performance (Bevis & Krulik, 1991). Education does not encourage unquestioning compliance with established procedures. In an educational environment, the teacher and student view one another as colleagues who share goals for the welfare of patients/clients.

There are also differences in the way one goes about training and educating. Bevis and Krulik (1991) have developed a schema of different learning types. Three of these are predominantly used in training and are the focus of technical learning programs. These are item learning, directive learning, and rationale learning.

Item learning is used in order to memorize the names of certain pieces of equipment used in a nursing procedure, their location on the unit, etc. *Directive learning* is used for instructing the execution of a procedure. The reasons for the procedure and the principles behind the procedure are called *rationale learning*. The rationale is needed to link theoretical knowledge to practice. This type of learning, however, is often missed when didactic instruction is separated from clinical experiences, as was characteristic of many nursing education programs in Central and Eastern Europe in the past and still persists in some parts of the world.

A second group of learning types—syntactical, contextual, and inquiry learning—are based on students' own learning and experiences, although not in a predetermined hierarchical sequence. The arrangement of data into logical structures of meaningful wholes is characteristic of syntactical learning. For those who are technically expert, any learning can be changed into *syntactical learning*. Syntactical learning involves consequential reasoning. It helps us to understand how theories, concepts and ideas are connected in practical usage (Bevis & Krulik, 1991). The foundations for syntactical learning are laid in university-level programs, but such learning is fully attained only after the learner has acquired some clinical expertise, since syntactical learning is experience-based and requires both theoretical knowledge and clinical experience. An example of such learning is the intuitive leap a nurse can make, after observing a sign or symptom, foregoing the usual procedure of verification of the observation, and proceeding with the necessary intervention.

Contextual learning deals with the interrelated conditions of the context in which nursing practice occurs (Bevis & Krulik, 1991). It pertains to the sociocultural context of nursing, the ways of being a nurse in a particular healthcare culture. It involves socialization into the profession and learning the relationships of the professional to patients/clients and to colleagues. It is learning the ways of being a professional nurse who is compassionate and caring and who uses nursing knowledge as the basis of actions in caring for individuals as well as influencing health care policy.

Inquiry learning is the mode of learning most important for the creation of science and the future of practice. According to Bevis and Krulik, it is the art of investigation, the search for truth, the generation of theory (1991). A curriculum at the university level must contain ample opportunities for this type of learning. It represents the creative aspect of the profession and is necessary in order to develop new strategies, to leap into new ways of conceptualizing. Inquiry learning allows students to discover their own meaning of nursing. They must have opportunities to observe the effects of their nursing care, search for answers to questions they encounter in practice, and contemplate the implications of viewing clinical phenomena from different perspectives. The problem-based educational method fosters inquiry learning. The use of knowledge from the humanities and arts in the study of nursing fosters the development of students' imagination and creativity and promotes inquiry learning.

In many countries of the world changes in political and economic structures, as well as changes in health care systems, have occurred at an exponential rate during the second half of this century. These changes provide many opportunities for the development of nursing. All over the world societies are requiring nursing care by educated nurses who attend to clients as human beings. In response to this need, the education of nurses is being moved to higher levels of the educational hierarchy, where it is possible to prepare nurses to develop both the science of nursing and nursing practice for the next millennium.

THE CRITICAL FACTOR

The critical link between curriculum design and the outcome of the curricular process is the nurse educator, both in the classroom and in clinical settings. Nurse educators constantly reshape the curriculum as they present content designed to achieve a certain goal. Teachers put their personal stamp on the curriculum. If their goal for education is merely the acquisition of the knowledge and skills required to practice nursing, without regard to what nursing is and who nurses are in relation to their patients/clients, all the structural intentions of a curriculum are for naught. Through their methods of teaching and their relationships with students, teachers convey their beliefs about the importance of the development of nursing as a profession, about nursing science and the importance of science-based practice, and about the importance of continually seeking new answers for questions encountered in practice.

Educators talk about the knowledgeable doer (Schoen, 1987) as the goal of nursing education. This knowledgeable doer is a person who is involved, who thinks, who does, and who uses the self in the care of patients/clients and thus creates the practice of today as well as the practice of the future. The new approach to teaching therefore must focus on the holistic development of every student, intellectually and interpersonally. This means taking the risk that nursing of the future will be quite different from what educators now envision. It may mean that nursing of the future will be molded by the nurses whom today's educators have encouraged to discover their present and future practice for themselves, through the development of nursing knowledge.

To summarize, then, the development of a nursing education curriculum that meets the needs both of science and of professional practice requires that both practice and the science of practice are viewed in the context where both occur. The curriculum provides only the structure for the process of education. Most important is the educator's attention to the learner's development—to the development of a person who practices in the here and now and will create the future knowledge base of the practice through inquiry.

> Whatever else education may set out to achieve it is its contribution to "the development of persons" which may be seen as its final justification. What is sometimes referred to as "individual personal development" becomes the final imperative and beyond that nothing need be said. To challenge it would be unthinkable. (Lawson, 1989, p. 95)

REFERENCES

Bevis, E. M. (1988). New directions for a new age. In E. M. Bevis (Ed.), *Curriculum revolution: Mandate for change*. New York: National League for Nursing.

Bevis, E. M., & Krulik, T. (1991). Nationwide faculty development: Model for a shift from diploma to baccalaureate education. *Journal of Advanced Nursing, 16*, 362–370.

Fitzpatrick, J. J., & Abraham, I. L. (1988). Toward the socialization of scholars and scientists. *Nurse Educator, 12*, 23–25.

Haase, P. T. (1990). *The origins and rise of associate degree nursing education*. New York: National League for Nursing.

Lawson, K. H. (1989). *Philosophical concepts and values in adult education*. (rev. ed.). Milton Keynes, London: Open University Press.

Oakeshott, M. (1989). *The voice of liberal learning*. New Haven, CT: Yale University Press.

Schoen, D. (1987). *Educating the reflective practitioner*. San Francisco: Jossey-Bass.

CHAPTER 6

Research on Teaching Methods in Nursing

Geraldine McCarthy, RGN, RNT, MED, MSN, PhD

TEACHING GROUPS: THE LECTURE AS A PEDAGOGICAL METHOD

Lecturing is the most frequently used teaching strategy and is used extensively for the education of large groups of students in both general and nursing education. The lecture is dependent on a deductive attitude. The teacher defines concepts, illustrating them with examples and unfolding the implications, and usually finishes by having the students make links with previously learned material. The lecture is a teacher-centered approach to education. It is a method of teaching which allows the teacher to exert control over the learning situation. It is argued by a number of authors (Freire, 1970; Heron, 1989) that, in such circumstances, the students are less able to direct their own learning or to think critically. They are thereby subjected to a passive, subservient role. It is argued that nurse education has traditionally been pedagogical in orientation (Pinkney, 1983) and dominated by the medical model (Hurst, 1985). It may therefore be judged as failing to treat students as adult learners and thus as an inappropriate educational strategy for the caring professions. However, educators who ascribe to the view that mental discipline enhances learning by developing the "faculties of the mind" favor the lecture.

There is no doubt that models of nurse education influence teaching strategies. In recent years many countries, including the United Kingdom, Australia, and Canada, have examined and altered their systems of nurse education and training from a hospital-based model to a third-level education-based model. In effect, this has major implications for teaching methods and student-teacher relationships. However, in many other countries throughout Europe, apprenticeship-type training, with the student nurse occupying a dual role as learner and employee, is still prevalent. The system means that students receive "blocks" of instruction in school and then function as both workers and learners in hospital wards. The student nurse is therefore exposed to potential teaching and learning situations in two quite separate and distinct environments: the school of nursing and the clinical areas of a hospital. Teaching methods in these two systems of education determine the learning done by students of nursing and the effectiveness of such learning.

The most common method of teaching apprentice-type student nurses is the lecture. Nursing students in universities are also taught predominantly by lecture, and at conferences on nursing throughout the world the lecture is the most common method of imparting information. It is asserted that this mechanism of teaching prepares students as passive members of a homogeneous group (Gott, 1982). Chittick (1968), in highlighting problems with the apprenticeship system of nurse training in Australia, argued that "No other group of young people in modern society receives such a narrow, restrictive and unimaginative type of education. Nurse education has few of the hallmarks of professional education" (p. 32). Research on lecturing revealed it to provoke criticisms of dependence (Davis, 1983, 1990; Jarvis, 1983) with the facts from the lecturer's notes flowing through the student's head and on to his note pad without interpretation or integration. Further, it is proposed that many educational programs require students to unquestionably follow the educational process designed for them by their teachers (Beard, 1978; Davis, 1983). In relation to any commitment to autonomy in learning in continuing education, Alexander (1983, 1984) suggested that it is undermined by earlier nursing experience of learning as a passive process resulting from "spoon feeding" and teachers' insistence on covering the curriculum.

However, lecturing is still the most popular teaching method (Satterfield, 1978) for large groups of students and is said to have many advantages (De Tornyay & Thompson, 1987). Research showed that the good lecturer is better than written material but the degree of learning, understanding, and integration depends on the communication skills of the lecturer (Foley & Smilansky, 1980; McKeachie, 1978; Southin, 1984) and perhaps cognitive congruence of student/teachers in terms of preference (Waltz, 1978) and values (Williams, Block, & Blair, 1978).

But what do students think? Research has focused on teaching by lecture compared with teaching by group discussion (Burnard & Morrisson, 1992) or with multiple teaching strategies There is some evidence that students prefer the traditional strategies of drill or recitation and concrete teacher-structured learning experiences (Ferrell, 1978; Garity, 1985; Ostmoe, Van Hoozen, Scheffel, & Crowell, 1984; Rezler & French, 1975). In a more recent study Vaughan (1990) found that students preferred methodologies that were student-centered. In studies (Burnard & Morrison, 1992; Ostmoe et al., 1984) where both teachers and students were requested to indicate preferred styles of teaching, it was found that baccalaureate students tended to prefer a teacher-centered approach to teaching which was highly organized, while the lecturers preferred a student-centered approach. Students of allied health professions showed similar attitudes (Rezler & French, 1975).

However, it is true that the results of studies on the lecture are inconclusive, possibly because in the research the outcome measures were ill-defined and difficult to measure. Further, bias may have been introduced in many of the studies while students were subjects to a number of teaching methods and then tested and where the teacher was both instructor and investigator. It appears that the lecture is effective if it is for reasons of imparting information for the minimum of effort to the maximum audience (Jones, 1990). However, there is evidence that other methods of teaching are more effective when teaching affective or attitudinal changes (Selby & Tuttle, 1985).

Teaching by Seminar and Guided Design

Other less used but equally group-oriented methods of teaching are the seminar and guided design. In the seminar, the student takes the initiative, but the discussion is guided by the teacher. The discussion involves the sharing of information and diverse ideas and recognizes the student as a participant in teaching. It has been said that this method of teaching promotes a deep understanding of learning as well as attitudes, interests and interpersonal relationships (Lowman, 1984). However, teachers who view education as information-giving and -receiving may not find discussion of much value. There is some research (Kramer, Holaday & Hoeffer, 1981) to show that small group work for teaching research was most effective at both graduate and undergraduate levels in relation to the development of attitudes.

Guided design is a problem-focused teaching mechanism. The teacher prepares problem-solving formats which the students use as a opportunity for decisionmaking. The student is thus helped to define problems, generate alternative solutions, and consider responses (Wales & Hageman, 1979). Advantages are listed as enthusiasm, motivation and excitement about learning, increased retention of information, and students' recognition that problems do not have neat answers. Disadvantages include intensive group situations, which some students dislike, and difficulty for teachers in constructing a guided design package, which is very time-consuming (De Tornyay & Thompson, 1987). Selby and Tuttle (1985) compared the attitudes of two groups of nursing students studying research in Masters'-level programs. They found that the students using guided design were significantly more positive in their attitudes to research and had higher post-test scores than the students being taught by more traditional methods.

As is true of the lecture method, there is very limited research investigating the use of either the seminar or guided design as teaching strategies. The results of studies comparing these methods of teaching with other methods are inconclusive, possibly because outcome measures were ill-defined and difficult to measure.

TEACHING INDIVIDUALS:
STUDENT-CENTERED TEACHING
ANDRAGOGICAL EDUCATION

Those who advocate (Knowles, 1978; Maslow, 1971; Rogers, 1969, 1983) breaking away from the teacher-dominated classroom in order to increase student participation and to cater to individual differences prescribe individualized teaching. Pedagogical difficulties can be controlled with the learner-centered approach and the introduction of self-directed learning and democratic procedures. The ideology of student-centered education is based on a theory of natural enfoldment and learning through a stimulating environment and a move towards increasing personal autonomy in determining what should be learned and how, according to individual needs. The philosophical model of education sustains the personal and professional growth of students. The outcome of such education is proposed as being critical analytical and reflective thinkers.

Many teaching strategies have been introduced as student-centered or nondirective. Included are methods such as interactive television, computerization, simulation, games and role playing, self-directed learning, contract learning, negotiated time, and experimental learning. The use of these in the acquisition of interpersonal skills, clinical problem-solving techniques, patient management problems, decisionmaking, development of awareness and sensitivity, and crisis intervention skills have been described in the literature (Donaldson, 1992; Selvin & Lavery, 1991; Whittaker, 1984). However, it is significant to note that Melia (1983) found that student nurses held the impression that the ideal image of a nurse to aim for is one who can cope, knows all the answers, and is always efficient; they found difficulty in admitting that they did not know something.

Much has been written on the strategies of teaching (Iwasiw, 1987; Slevin & Lavery, 1991), but what of the research effectiveness? Available research comparing individualized with traditional methods of teaching show individualized methods to be superior in relation to test scores (Foley & Smilansky, 1980, Southin, 1984), failure rates in examinations (Bitzer & Boudreaux, 1969; Timpke & Janney, 1981) and preferred method of learning (Kirchhoff & Holzemer, 1979; Neil, 1985; Van Dongan & Van Dongan, 1984).

Computerization

Computers have been used extensively in health care for information generation and dispersal, and in a few colleges they are used for computer-assisted learning (CAL). There are, of course, many nurses in many countries who have not had the opportunity to study via this method. Research on the effectiveness of CAL is sparse and that which is available compares CAL with traditional teaching methods. The results showed significant differences in terms of post-test scores for diploma test students in relation to describing care for patients with myocardial infarction and angina (Bitzer, 1966). This early study was supported by the findings of Bitzer and Boudreaux (1969) when teaching a course in maternity nursing; for Timpke and Janney (1981) when teaching drug dose calculations and Kirchhoff and Holzemer (1979) with baccalaureate students in relation to post-operative care. However, researchers have also found no significant differences between the test scores of students using computers and those using traditional learning methods (Conklin, 1983; Day & Payne, 1984). Although there is some conflicting evidence as to the effectiveness of the computer in teaching, it does appear that it is an overall effective individual teaching method. Learning with the computer may take less time, and retention of material may be improved. Further, computers have been found to be the preferred method of learning in a number of studies with undergraduate students (Kirchhoff & Holzemer, 1979; Neil, 1985; Van Donegan & Van Donegan, 1984; Warner & Tenney, 1985).

Using Simulation and Games

Using simulation and games has been advocated as an individual paced teaching and learning method. These methods became popular in the 1960s, and are thought of as having the potential to bring theory and real life experiences closer together. Models and simulation are commonly used in teaching nurses. For example: models for resuscitation, intravenous injection models which may be used for venipuncture skill acquisition, use of robots in medical learning, use of clinical laboratory, roleplaying to gain insight into the feelings of others and for learning interpersonal skills, and problem-solving and crisis intervention skills. Simulations are used, for example, by having students spend 24 hours in a wheelchair or blindfolded in an effort to gain insight into what it feels like to be immobilized or blind. Although there are many reports in the literature describing these methods of education (De Bella-Baldigo, 1984; Horn & Cleaves, 1980; Jeffers & Christensen, 1979; Kolb, 1983; Sim-Ed, 1978; Ulione, 1983) there are few which investigate their effectiveness. However, those that do exist provided support for the use of the various strategies in relation to learning attitudes and skills (Parathian & Taylor, 1993) affective and/or cognitive gains (Godejohn, Taylor, Muhlenkamp, & Blaesser, 1975; Holzemer, Schleutermann, Farrand, & Millar, 1981; Shaffer & Pfeiffer, 1980). Other researchers reported greater sensitivity towards mental patients after a period of being taught by using a simulation situation (Laszlo & McKenzie, 1979), and in attitudes towards mental patients (Goldejohn et al., 1975). One study (McLaughlin, Carr, & Delucchi, 1981) was found which examined the measurement properties of existing clinical simulation tests.

From a general education perspective, an analysis of the data available on simulation and games done by Bredemeier and Greenblat (1981) showed that there was some evidence to support the notion that these methods are as effective as other methods in teaching and learning in the cognitive and affective domains and that these methods may be useful for some but not all students. There is, however, little empirical evidence to support the contention that simulation has advantages over traditional teaching methods in nurse education. Difficulties with comparing research results are in relation to definition of terms and the differentiation of simulation from games. There is therefore a necessity for continuing research regarding student favorability, teaching methods, and outcome realization in relation to the use of the individual teaching strategies of simulations and games.

Individual Instruction and Decision Trees

While there have been numerous articles on teaching problem-solving and clinical judgment (Broderick & Ammentorp, 1979; Corcoran, 1986; Pyles & Stern, 1983; Smith & Russell, 1991; Westfall, Tanner, Putzier, & Patrick, 1986) and of successful methods of teaching (Farrand, Holzemer, & Schleutermann, 1982; McGuire, Solomen, & Bashook, 1975), there have been very few researchers who have systematically evaluated strategies for the teaching of clinical judgment and the advantages of such methods. Both Aspinal (1976) and Hamdi and Hutelmyer (1970) used an experimental design and explored the use of a decision tree and a structured assessment guide to identify patient problems and improve nursing diagnosis competency. For Aspinal (1976) the experimental group used problem-centered records and performed significantly better than the control group (using charting). For Hamdi and Hutelmeyer (1970) there was no difference between control and experimental groups on the ability of patient problems identification.

In two other studies of varying design, Mitchell and Atwood (1975) and Tanner (1982) examined the effectiveness of teaching methods on clinical judgment abilities of students. No significant effects were found. However, the teaching methods and outcome measures were diverse, leading to difficulties with comparison of results. In a study (Harvey & Vaughan, 1990) on student nurses' attitudes towards different teaching/learning methods, the researchers investigated the attitudes held by 203 students toward 10 different teaching methods which were categorized as either teacher-centered or student-centered. Findings were that discovery learning did not attract particularly favorable attitudes. This may have been due to the fact that in many discovery teaching strategies the student works alone, which is not always the student's preferred method of learning. In the study the teaching methods chosen as most favorable were those which were student-centered but involved groups of students. Overall, these few studies have results which are discouraging, particularly as it is stated that nurse education not only fails to stimulate critical thinking but actually stifles creativity and originality of thinking in student nurses (Elsemann, 1972) through the educational methods employed.

It appears that much more research is necessary on methods of teaching clinical judgment and on the effectiveness of individualized teaching strategies in the development of clinical judgment skills.

Experiential Learning

A major component of nurse education has always been the clinical experience in client settings in which nurses derive knowledge about nursing. Learning from experience or teaching/learning nursing where it is carried out is thought by many nurses to be the most effective method. Bradshaw (1978) concluded that most students in nursing programs are of the "*sensing-feeling*" type, who perceive the world more clearly through the use of the five senses, thus achieving the greatest learning benefit through involvement in concrete experiences.

Research has found that students see experiential learning in terms of clinical learning (Burnard, 1992) and describe learning in the clinical setting as that in "the real world"—learning by doing and by being involved in what was happening—as opposed to the traditional methods of learning.

Cognitive Style and Teaching/Learning

There is a great amount of research to support the assertion that each student learns in a way which is different from the next student (Kolb, 1983). Witkin (1973) has asserted that cognitive style is a potent variable in academic choice, and in how teachers teach and learning takes place. Laschainger (1984) found that concrete learning styles were more prevalent in the Majority of the 268 undergraduate students tested by the Kolb Learning Style Inventory. The sample comprised incoming and advanced students and suggested that perhaps nursing as a career attracted more concrete-oriented individuals, and that the learning style was accentuated by an increased exposure to the discipline of nursing. The results supported an earlier study (Christianson, Lee, & Bugg, 1979) that proposed that nurses need structured concrete experiences, as they may learn best in environments which involve direct experiences. This also was supported by O'Kell (1988) who studied preferences in one health district. However, Dux (1989) found that 119 students did not show a strong preference for any one learning style, but demonstrated a wide range and combination of preferred learning styles. In a 1972 study, Lange determined that the failure-withdrawal rate in specific nursing courses was lower when teachers and students were matched on learning style than when teachers and students were not matched. For Osbourne and Thompson (1977) open-minded students (as determined by Rokeach's Dogmatism Scale) achieved a significantly higher mean post-test score on learning modules than did their closed-minded peers. Thus, the closed-minded student benefitted less from the use of this independent learning strategy.

A number of studies have been focused on the effectiveness on learning of a variety of teaching methods in research programs. While a number of researchers (Austin, Opie, & Frazier, 1987; Broom & Demi, 1987; Davis, 1990; Perry, 1986; Warner & Tenney, 1985) reported positive findings, the findings are not supported empirically. Merritt (1983), when comparing generic and RN students on the basis of age and length of career employment, found that these factors did not account for differences in learning preferences. Other researchers explored the effects of a research course on cognitive development (Sakalys, 1984) and attitudes towards research before, during, and after a research course (Swanson & Kleinbaum, 1984). In both studies little difference was found as a result of teaching. Selby and Tuttle (1985) investigated knowledge and attitude to research after teaching a research course which focused on learning styles and reported a positive change in attitude after the course.

These studies require replication with large groups entering nursing, as knowledge concerning the preferred ways of learning of nursing students may be useful in the selection of teaching strategies. Kolb (1976) suggested that students learn best when teaching matches their learning styles. De Tornyay (1983) called for continuing research on the topic of teaching-learning to ensure that curricular developments are in line with requirements and are based on empirical knowledge rather than fashion. Certainly, there is a lack of support for the full-scale use of nontraditional strategies with all students. Perhaps we should ask instead "Which method is most useful for an individual student at a particular stage of development?" and "Which method is best for the subject matter and desired outcomes?" From an educational perspective, student attitudes, particularly students' educational attitudes, should be a major concern of teachers, because the primary goals of teachers should include the development of positive educational attitudes.

CONCLUSIONS

Based on the literature reviewed, there is still a widespread use of lectures in nursing education. Other teaching strategies focusing on the individual are also used in nurse education, and theory says that they are effective, especially in relation to the development of attitudes, skills, and problem-solving abilities. Overall, the research on teaching methods showed that many nurses and nursing students prefer direct, concrete, teacher-structured experiences; and have a positive attitude to most teaching methods, both traditional and nontraditional but prefer highly organized activities with clearly stated requirements and expectations. However, it appears from the literature that there is a paucity of research on teaching methods in nursing. Most of the research done on teaching methods was done in the 1960s and 1970s and little research has been produced in the last decade. There appears to have been a shift towards clinical research by nurses and funding agencies throughout the world, to the detriment of nursing education research. Considerable thought should be given to the promotion of such research, because without it nurse educators will be devoid of research on teaching and learning and will be unable to determine the needs of students of nursing.

The increasingly complex demands made upon today's nurses in terms of technical, managerial, educational, and interpersonal expertise have been accompanied by calls on nurse educators to teach in a learner-centered way which fosters the development of critical thinking and self-direction in study. It is suggested that the vast increase in knowledge in nursing obliges educators to move away from an orientation of teaching facts and bits of information towards a more subject-centered approach and towards a student learning-centered approach.

There is an expanding body of nursing knowledge which has to be transmitted to students of nursing in diverse situations throughout the world. Many students live in areas far removed from college facilities and the possibility of educating these individuals at home or in centers far removed from colleges offers the challenge of finding alternatives to traditional methods of educating. There is, therefore, a great importance in evaluating different methods of teaching, as it behooves teachers to know the strategies that are most effective.

Students are rarely assessed for their individual learning skills, and rarely are a multiplicity of teaching methods offered to match cognitive choice. Seldom are nursing students permitted to take a different route from other students in their learning. Perhaps what is necessary is for teachers to choose a variety of teaching methods based on the characteristics of both the learners and students.

REFERENCES

Alexander, M. F. (1984). Learning to nurse: Beginning has implications for continuing. *Nurse Education Today, 4,* 4–7.

Alexander, M. F. (1983). *Learning to nurse: Integrating theory and practice*. Edinburgh: Churchill Livingstone.

Aspinall, M. J. (1976). Nursing diagnosis: The weak link. *Nursing Outlook, 24*, 433–437.

Austin, J. K., Opie, N. D., & Frazier, H. A. (1987). Strategy for teaching evaluation research in psychiatric/mental health nursing. *Journal of Nursing Education, 26*, 108–112.

Bitzer, M. (1966). Clinical nursing instruction via the PLATO simulated laboratory. *Nursing Research, 15*, 144–150.

Bitzer, M. D., & Boudreaux, M. C. (1969). Using a computer to teach nursing. *Nursing Forum, 8*, 234–254.

Bradshaw, S. (1978). Concentrated experiential learning laboratories. *Journal of Nursing Education, 17*, 32–35.

Bredemeier, M. E., & Greenblat, C. S. (1981). The educational effectiveness of simulation games: A synthesis. In C. S. Greenblat & R. D. Duke (Eds.), *Principles and practices of gaming-simulation* (pp. 285–291). Beverly Hills, CA: Sage.

Broderick, M. E., and Ammentorp, W. (1979). Information structures: An analysis of nursing performance. *Nursing Research, 28*, 106–110.

Broome, M. E., & Demi, A. S. (1987). Strategies for teaching nursing research: Teaching statistical analysis: A computer application activity. *Western Journal of Nursing Research, 9*, 132–137.

Burnard, P. (1992). Student nurses' perceptions of experiential learning. *Nurse Education Today, 12*, 163–173.

Burnard, P., & Morrisson, P. (1991). Students and lecturers preferred teaching strategies. *International Journal of Nursing Studies, 29*, 345–353.

Chittick, R. (1968, April–June). Assignment report. New South Wales.

Christianson, M., Lee, P., & Bugg, P. (1979). Professional development of nurse practitioners as a function of need motivation, learning style and locus of control. *Nursing Research, 28*, 51–56.

Conklin, D. (1983). A study of computer assisted instruction in nursing education. *Journal of Computer Based Instruction, 9*, 98–107.

Corcoran, S. (1986). Planning by expert and novice nurses in cases of varying complexity. *Research in Nursing and Health, 9*, 155–162.

Davis, B. D. (1990). How nurses learn and how to improve the learning environment, *Nurse Education Today, 10*, 405–409.

Davis, B. D. (1983). *A Repertoire Gris Study of formal and informal aspects of student nurse training*. PhD Thesis, London University.

Day, R., & Payne, L. (1984). Comparison of lecture presentation versus computer managed instruction. In R. De Tornyay & M. Thompson (Eds.), *Strategies for teaching nursing* (p. 294). New York: Wiley.

De Bella-Baldigo, S. (1984). Fostering nurses' participation in health care planning. *Journal of Nursing Education, 23*, 124–125.

De Tornyay, R. (1983). Why nursing education research? *Journal of Nursing Education, 22*, 51.

De Tornyay, R., & Thompson, M. A. (1987). *Strategies for teaching nursing*. New York: Wiley.

Donaldson, I. (1992). The use of learning contracts in the clinical area. *Nurse Education Today, 12*, 431–436.

Dux, C. M. (1989). An investigation into whether nurse teachers take into account the individual learning styles of their students when formulating teaching strategies. *Nurse Education Today, 9*, 186–191.

Elsemann, R. (1972). Creativity in nursing students and their attitudes towards mental illness. *Journal of Clinical Psychology, 28*, 218–219.

Farrand, L., Holzemer, W. R., & Schleutermann, J. A. (1982). A study of construct validity simulation as a method of nurse practitioner problem-solving skills. *Nursing Research, 31*, 37–42.

Ferrell, B. (1978). Attitudes towards learning styles and self direction of ADN students. *Journal of Nursing Education, 17*, 19–22.

Foley, R. P., & Smilansky, J. (1980). *Teaching techniques: A handbook for health professionals*. New York: McGraw Hill.

Freire, P. (1970). *Pedagogy of the oppressed*. London: Penguin.

Garity, J. (1985). Learning styles: Basis for creating teaching and learning. *Nurse Educator, 10*, 12–16.

Godejohn, C. J., Taylor, J., Muhlenkamp, A. F., & Blaesser, W. (1975). Effect of simulation gaming on attitudes towards mental illness. *Nursing Research, 24*, 367–370.

Gott, M. (1982). Theories of learning and the teaching of nursing. *Nursing Times, 78*, 41–44.

Hamdi, M. E., & Hutelmyer, C. M. (1970). A study of the effectiveness of an assessment tool in the identification of nursing care problems. *Nursing Research, 19*, 354–359.

Harvey, T. J., & Vaughan, J. (1990). Student nurse attitude towards different teaching/learning methods. *Nurse Education Today, 10*, 181–185.

Heron, J. (1989). *Six category intervention analysis*. Guilford: University of Surrey.

Holzemer, W. L., Schleutermann, J. A., Farrand, L. L., & Millar, A. A. (1981). A validation study: Simulation as a measure of nurse practitioners' problem solving skills. *Nursing Research, 30*, 139–144.

Horn, R. E., & Cleaves, A. (Eds.). (1980). *The guide to simulation/games for education and training*. Beverly Hills: Sage.

Hurst, K. (1985). Traditional versus progressive nurse education: A review of the literature. *Nurse Education Today, 5*, 30–35.

Iwasiw, C. I. (1987). The role of the teacher in self directed learning. *Nurse Education Today, 7*, 222–227.

Jarvis, P. (1983). *Professional education*. London: Croom Helm.

Jeffers, J. M., & Christensen, M. G. (1979). Using simulation to facilitate the acquisition of clinical observational skills, *Journal of Nursing Education, 18*, 29–32.

Jones, R. G. (1990). The lecture as an education method in modern nurse education. *Nurse Education Today, 10*, 290–293.

Kirchhoff, K. T., & Holzemer, W. (1979). Student learning and a computer-assisted instructional program. *Journal of Nursing Education, 18*, 22–30.

Knowles, M. (1978). *The adult learner: A neglected species*. Houston: Gulf Publishing.

Kolb, S. E. (1983). A game for teaching concepts of patient care. *Nurse Educator, 8*(3), 84–86.

Kramer, M., Holaday, R., & Hoeffer, B. (1981). The teaching of nursing research. Part II: A comparison of teaching strategies. *Nurse Educator, 6*, 30–37.

Lange, C. (1972). Autotutorial techniques nursing education. Englewood Cliffs, NJ: Prentice-Hall.

Laschanger, A. H. (1984). Learning styles of nursing students and career choices. *Journal of Advanced Nursing, 9*, 375–380.

Laszlo, S. S., & McKenzie, J. L. (1979). The use of a simulation game in training hospital staff about patients' rights. *Journal of Continuing Education in Nursing* 10, 30, 35–36.

Lowman, J. (1984). *Mastering the techniques of teaching*. San Francisco: Jossey Bass.

Maslow, A. (1971). *The further reaches of human nature*. London: Penguin.

McGuire, C. H., Solomen, L. M., & Bashook, P. G. (1975). *Construction and use of written simulation*. New York: Psychological Corporation.

McKeachie, W. J. (1978). *Teaching tips: Guidebook for the beginning college teacher*. Lexington, MA: Heath.

McLaughlin, F. E., Carr, J., & Delucchi, K. (1981). Measurement properties of clinical simulation tests: Hypertension and chronic obstructive pulmonary disease. *Nursing Research, 30*, 5–9.

Melia, K. (1983). Students' views of nursing. *Nursing Times, 79*, 24–27.

Merritt, S. (1983). Learning style preferences of baccalaureate nursing students. *Nursing Research, 32*, 367–372.

Mitchell, P. H., & Atwood, J. (1975). Problem-oriented recording as a teaching learning tool. *Nursing Research, 24*, 99–103.

Neil, R. M. (1985). Effects of computer assisted instruction on nursing student learning and attitude. *Journal of Nursing Education, 24*, 74–75.

O'Kell, S. P. (1988). A study of the relationship between learning style, readiness for self directed learning and teaching preferences of learner nurses in one health district. *Nurse Education Today, 8*, 197–204.

Osbourne, W. P., & Thompson, M. A. (1977). Variables associated with student mastery of learning modules. In M. V. Batey (Ed.), *Communicating nursing research* (Vol. 9) (167–180). Boulder, CO: Western Interstate Commission for Higher Education.

Ostmoe, P., Van Hoozen, H., Scheffel, A., & Crowell, C. (1984). Learning style preference and selection of learning strategies: Considerations and implications for nurse educators. *Journal of Nurse Education, 23*, 27–30.

Parathian, A. R., & Taylor, F. (1993). Can we insulate trainee nurses from exposure to bad practice: A study of role play in communicating bad news to patients. *Journal of Advanced Nursing, 18*, 801–807.

Perry, P. A. (1986). Strategies for teaching nursing research: Integration of research in a graduate clinical course. *Western Journal of Nursing Research, 8*, 124–127.

Pinkney, V. J. (1983). Nursing education as adult education: A philosophical standpoint. *Curationis, 6*, 8–10.

Pyles, S. H., & Stern, P. N. (198). Discovery of nursing gestalt in critical care nursing: The importance of the grey gorilla syndrome. *Image: The Journal of Nursing Scholarship, 15*, 51–57.

Rezler, A. G., & French, R. M. (1975). Personality types and learning preferences of students in six allied health professions. *Journal of Allied Health, 4*, 20–26.

Rogers, C. (1969). *Freedom to learn.* Columbus, OH: Merrill.

Rogers, C. (1983). *Freedom to learn for the eighties.* Columbus, OH: Merrill.

Sakalys, J. A. (1984). Effects of an undergraduate research course on cognitive development. *Nursing Research, 33*, 290–295.

Satterfield, J. (1978). Lecturing. In O. Milton (Ed.), *On college teaching* (pp. 34–61). San Francisco: Jossey Bass.

Selby, M. L., & Tuttle, D. M. (1985). Teaching nursing research by guided design: A pilot study. *Journal of Nursing Education, 24*, 250–295.

Shaffer, M. K., & Pfeiffer, I. L. (1980). You too can prepare videotapes for instruction. *Journal of Nursing Education, 19*, 23–27.

Sim-Ed. (1978). *Catalog of educational simulation.* Tucson, Arizona: The University of Arizona, College of Education.

Slevin, O. D., & Lavery, M. C. (1991). Self directed learning and student supervision. *Nurse Education Today, 11*, 368–377.

Smith, A., & Russell, J. (1991). Using critical learning incidents in nurse education. *Nurse Education Today, 11*, 284–294.

Southin, J. L. (1984). Inquiry and explanation in introductory science. In K. I. Spear (Ed.), *Rejuvenating introduction courses* (pp. 99–108). San Francisco: Jossey Bass.

Swanson, I., & Kleinbaum, A. (1984). Attitude towards research among undergraduate nursing students. *Journal of Nursing Education, 23*, 380–386.

Tanner, C. A. (1982). Instruction in the diagnostic process: An experimental study. In M. Kim & D. Moritz (Eds.), *Classification of nursing diagnosis: Proceedings of the third and fourth national conference* (pp. 145–152). New York: McGraw Hill.

Timpke, J., & Janney, C. P. (1981). Teaching drug dosage by computer. *Nursing Outlook, 29*, 376–377.

Ulione, M. S. (1983). Simulation gaming in nurse education. *Journal of Nursing Education, 22*, 349–351.

Van Dongen, C. J., & Van Dongen, W. O. (1984). Using microcomputers to teach psychopharmacology. *Journal of Nursing Education, 23*, 259–260.

Vaughan, T. A. Student nurse attitudes to teaching/learning methods, *Journal of Advanced Nursing, 15*, 925–933.

Wales, S. K., & Hageman, V. (1979). Guided design systems approach in nursing education. *Journal of Nursing Education, 18*, 38–45.

Waltz, C. F. (1978). Faculty influence on nursing students' preferences for practice. *Nursing Research, 24*, 89–97.

Warner, S., & Tenney, J. W. (1985). Strategies for teaching nursing research: A test of computer-assisted instruction in teaching nursing research. *Western Journal of Nursing Research, 7*, 132–134.

Whittaker, A. F. (1984). Use of contract learning. *Nurse Educator Today*, 36–39.

Williams, M. A., Block, D. W., & Blair, E. M. (1978). Values and value changes of graduate nursing students: Their relationship to faculty values and to selected educational factors. *Nursing Research, 27*, 181–189.

Witkin, H. A. (1973). *The role of cognitive style in academic performance and in teacher student relations*. Princeton, NJ: Educational Testing Service.

Westfall, M. E., Tanner, C. A., Putzier, D. K., & Patrick, K. P. (1986). Clinical reference in nursing: A preliminary analysis of cognitive strategies. *Research in Nursing and Health, 9,* 269–277.

CHAPTER 7

Some Thoughts on the Art of Teaching Nursing

Brigitta Hochenegger-Haubmann

T eaching basically means giving methodical instruction in a certain subject, and thus requires critical incorporation and systematization. In addition, teaching also includes emotional and social experience and behavior, since there is a continual interaction between teacher and pupil and between pupil and pupil. Thus, teaching plays an essential part in education.

The main emphases of lessons vary according to the different types of schools. Nursing education includes vocational training; one of its aims is to offer both theoretical and practical preparation for the job. Therefore, the most important forms of giving lessons in this type of school are teaching and instructing. These two forms are complementary in that teaching provides the theory, whereas instructing is a methodical, systematic approach to practice. Due to this complex framework of interrelations and effects, teaching also includes a more or less important imponderable, which can be dealt with only by spontaneity; thus it seems to be justified to speak of teaching as an art.

In a critical review of the role of teaching in nursing it is important to define nursing and its purpose.

Nursing is an independent profession and a separate part of the health services. Nurses determines the extent of the need for nursing care and are responsible for the planning, carrying out, and evaluation of care as well as for training and further education. Nursing training has a scientific basis of its own and makes use of the findings of medicine, natural sciences, the humanities, and social sciences. Care is concerned with both healthy and sick people and thus also involves preventive measures. Care is oriented to the person's individual needs; the patient should be treated in a holistic way. Various theories and models of nursing offer holistic approaches. In holistic care, the patient is seen as a partner whose dignity and rights are respected and whose autonomy is maintained and encouraged.

In order to come up to the requirements in nursing, teaching has to fulfill the following tasks:

59

- it should impart to students not only general and job-related knowledge, but also practical skills,
- it should help students develop a sense of social and professional responsibility, and
- it should support the students' personal development by teaching them constructive criticism, flexibility, and respect for the individual's dignity and rights.

This sounds all very good. We all want to fulfill these tasks, of course. However, the question arises as to whether teaching in nursing can meet all these expectations. How can we transform well-formulated theory into practical deeds?

In order to answer this question, an effort will be made to show if and how the various tasks can be translated into action and point to possible problems.

It is an important part of professional education to impart to students not only general and job-related knowledge, but also practical skills; after all, a good nurse is expected to know what she does, why and how.

Students are often confused by the great number of special, hardly differing methods of nursing and treatment. In practice, they often have difficulties in planning, justifying, carrying out, and evaluating the various measures individually. It is, therefore, very important to impart principles in teaching, and not to waste time with detailed knowledge and so burden students with "secondary, unnecessary knowledge."

Well-organized teaching material uses the knowledge of preclinical and clinical subjects as well as of natural and social sciences in order to answer questions concerning nursing care. Any kind of "miniature faculty of medicine" is not conducive to the interests of the profession.

Nursing schools should teach students to be responsible, constructive, flexible persons thinking for themselves, who respect a person's individuality, dignity, and rights. A mere presentation of endless strings of rules for dealing with patients is not appropriate.

Are personal development and individuality desired in nursing training? Do students experience for themselves personal care, tolerance and respect for the individual—things which they are expected to show later for their patients? The important task of conveying these goals and attitudes to students can most likely be realized by the teacher through use of various teaching and learning methods. For example,

- by consequently supporting projects;
- by encouraging various forms of self-experience;
- by using teaching methods related to situations and acting;

- by organizing learning by discovering and exercises suited to the brain; and
- by employing games, case studies and team teaching.

Literary texts can support the students' understanding and help eliminate the distance often caused by scientific texts. Literature can serve as a very good starting point for discussions. It offers possibilities for identification and can trigger off emotional reactions that might lead to real commitment.

These forms of learning, teaching, and instructing methods not only change the relationship between teacher and students but also the teacher's role. Instead of merely providing students with a wide range of information, there is a gradual movement to a student-centered, supportive learning method, thus facilitating the learning process. Students go through various stages of development: they carry out work, give advice, make choices, adapt themselves to new situations, and are finally able to develop something completely new. They develop from dependence to independence in order to finally be able to carry out executive duties.

Teachers experience learning with their students; they try to discover, do research, and live together. Teachers do not only act as mere lecturers and tutors teaching their students, but they also motivate them, do administrative work, organize social events, experiment and do research with their students, and sometimes even act as colleagues and friends.

In every professional education including nursing the relationship between theory and practice appears to be problematic. Nursing schools offer their students the possibility and the task of interrelating theory with practice by clinical teaching. It is this very form of teaching that may be the strong point of nursing education because neither "pure" theory nor mere instruction of practical skills can exist separately.

The art of teaching in nursing care is to show students the transfer from theory into practice, so that they can experience it for themselves. It is the task of teachers to reduce mutual prejudices and to establish a dialogue with the other side. It is important to create a good learning atmosphere and an individual fostering of students; this is possible only if all those involved in the training process are open to one another.

In each field of work, people must be able to plan, organize, and evaluate their own work and be responsible for its continuation. Nursing care as a separate field of knowledge with its own questions should be a matter of concern for all of us.

A good nursing school should provide good practice, together with efficient organization. Only in this way can high quality be guaranteed.

Establishing nursing care and nursing science at universities has considerable impact on the profession itself. This has become evident in countries already offering university training.

Nurse educators are often asked whether university education is necessary for good nursing care. After all, it is generally supposed that everything has worked well without university-trained staff. The demands in nursing care have become more complex and more intensive. In practice, in teaching and in management, holistic care requires nurses who are able to meet these demands. Above all, nursing care needs colleagues who are able to make contribution to the health service visible and measurable. The fear that graduate nurses might turn away from care is unfounded. Experience has shown that those who have acquired profound knowledge at university generally stay longer in care, and also longer in direct nursing care than less well-educated nurses.

CHAPTER 8

Teaching Nursing Research

Dott. Piera Poletti

Research is considered by the nursing scientific and professional community as the energy for development of the discipline. Through research the discipline's knowledge and instrumentation have increased. Moreover, the experience carried out in an area becomes, if validated, useful in many other contexts. Research has been widely considered an extremely important tool for the profession to: (a) increase knowledge within the discipline; (b) demonstrate the profession's value and potential; (c) highlight the social role of the profession; (d) provide professionals with new, more effective instruments; and (e) better connect education and practice. However, the linkage among the three areas of practice, education, and research has not been widely understood and actualized. Even if strong efforts are made by leaders of each area to emphasize the necessity of the connection, there are still many problems.

Nurses at different levels of education and roles are involved in three functions related to research: promoting, producing, and consuming research. As a consequence, research is considered an important element in the nursing curriculum, both at basic and advanced level. In a few countries research has been included in nursing curricula for many years, i.e. in the United States (Kovacs, 1974); in other countries, research has a short history of inclusion in nursing programs.

The first function, promoting research, requires responsibility of executives to look for funding. Also, researchers have to develop proposals and professionals have to identify problems in areas where there is lack of knowledge, where research has to be initiated. Even if promoting is primarily the researcher's task, executives and managers have to provide all the resources required and professionals have to cooperate in collecting data, and also in introducing changes in their own work.

Consuming research is a responsibility of everyone. However, nurses often choose to refer to their own experience instead of turning to the research literature. As a result, the care provided is not the most effective possible, and sometimes methods are not developed by a scientific approach or they are not updated. Assuming that to guarantee quality of care is not just "to do things we are able to do," even with passion, but "to provide the best possible care using knowledge available at the present time,'' every health care professional has to refer to literature and as a consequence has to introduce new methods and instruments into practice. This approach requires first of all a mentality oriented to research. Many factors are important in developing and guaranteeing the pursuit of this mentality by nurses: first, every professional nurse and every health care institution has the responsibility to provide clients with the best products in order to accomplish the institutional philosophy and purpose. However, the greatest responsibility to develop a research mentality and skills by nurses has to be attributed to the educational system, both at the basic and advanced levels, and through continuing education programs. This is why it is urgent to analyze and, if appropriate, modify the approach educational institutions utilize in developing attitudes toward research. In this chapter approaches to teaching research are introduced, also referring to international literature published between 1981 and the first half of 1993. A Medline search was conducted using the key words teaching, nursing, research, education, and program. The purposes of the paper are to present an approach to analyzing literature used in teaching research; communicate approaches introduced for teaching research; and highlight future development of teaching research methodology. The topic is presented referring to the following areas: research in nursing education; teaching research; and future developments.

RESEARCH IN NURSING EDUCATION

Education is the way to prepare professionals for the future. Thus, every decision about curricula has to be assumed to refer to the relevance of the content introduced to the work the professional has to implement. As the professional will be in the working world for many years, the perspective has to be the future needs of the society. Therefore, the future goals must be clear. A few elements can be cited to provide the coordinates for the future scenario: (a) A continuous change in health needs, including discovery of new diseases and reappearance of old diseases that we assumed had disappeared, but in fact had not; b) A troubled social scenario, where economic difficulties increase poverty, change social relationships, and require the ability to deal with different situations, and adapt to new ways of living; and c) Constant and increased technology development requiring skills to work with different facilities and supplies, to change procedures and methods.

As a consequence of these changes future professionals will be required to have: (a) a wide perspective on problems and situations; (b) flexibility; (c) ability to deal with complexity; and (d) the ability to learn continuously from not only their own experience, but also from literature. They need to be involved in developing organizational and technical change; thus, they have to be updated and able to participate in research programs (Poletti, 1993).

Generally speaking, objectives of a research course could be the following: (a) use research; (b) produce research; (c) collaborate in research projects; and (d) introduce research findings in professional practice.

Referring to the previous description of the connection between practice and research, there are different expectations from the different levels of educational programs including hospital-based programs; bachelor's degree programs; master's degree programs; doctoral programs, including the DNSc and the PhD; and continuing education. It has to be considered here that the situation is much different around the world: there are countries where education is based only in hospital settings, others where education is only at university level, and others where it is at both levels.

Professionals prepared at the undergraduate level are expected to identify researchable problems; gather data to refine practice; evaluate research reports; utilize findings from credible studies in their nursing practice; and share research findings with colleagues (American Nurses Association Commission on Nursing Research, 1981).

According to Overfield and Duffy (1984) nurses must be able to read critically research reports, judge the pertinence to patient care, and use findings of those judged to be adequately investigated. They need to be able to know when research findings are suited for adoption into their patient care repertoire. To guarantee an effective change in practice and in the discipline, even professional nurses prepared at the hospital level, especially in countries where it is the only way of education, have to be able to perform these tasks.

According to Firlit, Kemp, and Walsh (1986) master's-prepared professional nurses are expected to analyze critically; evaluate; and apply research in clinical practice. Doctorally prepared nurses have to design research projects; write research proposals; organize project implementation; conduct, direct, and supervise research implementation; elaborate, analyze, and interpret data; and report results. Continuing education programs have to pursue goals related to the actual level of professional practice in the research field required by the role assumed by the nurse participants. A needs assessment is the first step of any program development. From its results the other elements of the program have to be identified: objectives, contents, didactic activities and methods, human and instrumental resources, use of time, and evaluation criteria.

TEACHING RESEARCH

In order to analyze nursing literature related to teaching research, a grid is proposed. The following criteria were included:

(a) Purpose of the description of the reported material, including experience; research; and literature review;

(b) If it is research: quantitative approach used; qualitative approach used; both quantitative and qualitative approach used; relevance of the research; internal coherence of the research methodology utilized; correctness of methodology utilized; conclusions drawn; and implications for educational practice;

Also evaluated were the didactic act, including:

(a) Subjects the program was directed to (students or professionals; of varying levels of preparation such as: Bachelor's, Master's, Doctor of Nursing Science, Doctor of Philosophy;

(b) Objectives;

(c) Contents, especially research approach (quantitative or qualitative) taught;

(d) Didactic methodology used to teach research, including approach; strategy; setting; methods; instruments used/developed; and evaluation criteria;

(e) Results; and

(f) Recommendations.

An explanation is required for two of the terms used above: "approach" and "setting." Overfield and Duffy (1984) referred to the many ways to teach research and they categorized them into three main approaches: (a) learn by doing, e.g., students do an actual research study, (b) learn by proposing to do, e.g., students can be taught how to write a proposal but not be required to collect, analyze, or report the findings; and (c) learn by critiquing; students can be helped to read critically several research articles and as a final assignment to produce a scientific literature review on a topic of their choice. They also cited a more nebulous integrated approach, in which the instructor uses one or more of the three basic methods in varying degrees, without explaining it or presenting examples or support their negative judgement.

Abel and Sherman (1991) introduced a different way of realizing the "learn by doing" approach. The students were provided with a large national data set. They were requested to do a secondary data analysis, so they could complete part of the process related to doing research, without the effort required by collecting data. Poletti, Vinn, and Vittadello (1993) stated that the possibility for students to work with data and interpret results produced by their own work helps in developing interest toward research. Another integration of the "learn by doing" approach was suggested by Lee (1988) who proposed the meta-analysis method. Producing a meta-analysis, "students are exposed to all steps of the research process normally encountered in primary and secondary analysis and gain ample experience with statistical manipulation of data. Students using a meta-analysis approach complete their experience with a quantified conclusion and a clear sense of the direction in which their research should continue". (p. 33).

A consideration has to be given to a partial utilization of the "learn by doing" approach, considering in this category even the learning by doing just a part of the research process, such as data collection. In this case students experience a part of the research process, but not the insight in the connected consequential component. Therefore, they do not develop a complete perception of the process itself. This is supported also by Bzdek and Ganong (1986), who stated that "the student would be given at least some experience with each step, which is more important than the depth in which the process is taught" (p. 25).

An effective development of the "propose to do" approach was introduced by Selby and Tuttle (1985, 1988). They introduced "guided design," a didactic strategy developed in three steps. First, students learn basic concepts and principles; then they are assigned specific readings, exercises, and discussion, guided by an instructor's prepared study guide; the last step is the identification of a researchable problem and the development of a research proposal. In order to do so, a clinical situation is provided as a scenario where a role model (a hypothetical professional) faces problems requiring research to be solved; it is essential that the possibility exist for the student to identify with the described nurse. Research testing the use of this strategy at the Master's level, using a quasi-experimental design, described by the cited authors, provided evidence to support the usefulness of the approach, both for the development of knowledge and attitudes toward research.

A fourth approach can be identified to develop attitudes toward and knowledge about research, using research in teaching all the topics. Research has been identified by many programs as a thread throughout the curriculum, and faculty incorporate research findings in courses at all levels (Anderson, 1992). However, Poletti and Vian (1992) stated the core of the problem is the method by which research contents are provided. In fact, the expected impact can be achieved only if students are required to deal with all the other contents using a research approach. It means that they have to look at knowledge referring to the methods used to produce it, analyze problems following a research approach, and so on. Moreover, it is essential to provide research articles and books as didactic material for students. As far as possible, lessons and didactic activities have to be developed referring to research products and methodology. Spector and Bleeks (1980) suggested five teaching strategies that might aid integration: consistency, modelling, enthusiasm, clinical application, and a written assignment. They suggested the following: (a) stress the practical and clinical application of research; (b) do not overwhelm the students with too much research material; and (c) integrate research from the beginning of the nursing curriculum.

Using a pervasive approach based on research covering the complete curriculum, the 4 different approaches can be all used and integrated, pursuing a wide preparation in an acceptable amount of time. Students can become accurate readers using literature to study all the didactic contents, while on the other hand, they have the opportunity to develop a better understanding of the methodology by doing their own projects. Referring to the ANA (1981) requirements, through this experience students can learn: (a) how to deal with people and situations when they collect data collaborating in others' projects and when they have to introduce new approaches in their own practice; (b) to better understand the relationship between problems and knowledge, so to be able to identify "researchable" problems; (c) to analyze phenomena in order to evaluate the contents and the structure of the instruments used in research projects and articles; and (d) to experience the value of obtaining findings and presenting them to professionals. Moreover, they can be exposed to the obstacles to convince future colleagues to introduce changes in their own practice related to research findings.

Only by considering all the elements can students achieve all the objectives established by ANA (1981). The study carried out by Poletti et al. (1992, 1993) in seven Italian schools, involving 243 students along the 3-year nursing school program, supported the effectiveness of the approach. The prerequisite to the success of using this approach is a firm belief by the responsible school and availability of faculty to work together.

Many researchers have complained that a big problem with teaching research is the time. It has to be considered that the total amount of time for nursing programs is much different among countries and even schools. The 4610 hour program required by the European Community are not always comparable with other shorter programs. In this case also many hours are devoted to clinical practice (2850 in total); these could be used for research experience. However, with a pervasive approach, a better relationship between use of time and educational goals can be pursued.

Setting refers to the area in which students are required to apply their concepts and practice in order to learn research. Settings to be considered include: schools of nursing, classrooms and laboratories; clinical settings, hospital wards, community services; patients' homes; nursing homes and hospices; and communities, kindergarten, retirement homes, and workplaces. Types of assignments to be carried out in the classroom setting are: develop projects and proposals; secondary data analysis; meta-analysis; and critique of article. Applications in clinical and community settings aim to let students gain research experience. Students can be required to: (a) develop individual projects; and (b) collect data as assistants in research projects. This role is widely described by Gueldner, Clayton, Bramlett, & Boettcher (1993).

The same authors introduced incentives and recognition for students' research work through a monetary reimbursement or credits. Honors research projects (Woodtli, 1990) have been developed referring to the same criterion. However, there is not enough evidence to support the differential use of such incentives.

The concern of most authors was to develop positive attitudes toward research. This is consistent with the analysis described in the introduction. In fact, if research is not considered relevant for the clinical practice by professionals, tutors, and mentors, students who identify with them consider literature as a distant interest and not an important tool for their work. Referring to the topic, Gueldner et al. state: "It is imperative to find a way to excite our young students about research so that they will value it and include it as an integral part of their practice" (p. 18).

The effectiveness of a research course depends on many ingredients:

The strategy. This includes where, when, and how (methods and tools) the research is conducted.

The context. How is research considered in the school and in the clinical setting where students work? Through observing and learning from others values we develop our own values and attitudes. As stated by Gueldner et al., (1993):

> The subtle but critical ambience of scientific inquiry cannot be captured from readings and classroom activities. Just as one learns language best through purposeful use, nursing students can best learn the language of scholarship by engaging in scholarly communications with their faculty, and by observing them as role models. (p. 20)

The faculty. Teaching research requires research competence and didactic competence. If one of the two competencies is lacking, results are not as they could be. Often people who teach something have studied only through books; they much lack experience or enthusiasm. VanBree (1985) stated,

> Faculty who are enthusiastic about their subject are more likely to instill this enthusiasm into their students. Part of the ability to teach at a level appropriate to the baccalaureate student, is the ability to put research concepts into a black and white framework as much as possible. It is important that students learn the concepts in as concrete a manner as possible. (p. 85)

In other words, teachers rich in content but able just to speak for themselves, lose students' attention, and, as a consequence, their motivation and their learning. Molloy and Isaak (1989) stressed the fact that faculty must be creative in using their talents to direct the interest of students toward research. This requires teachers to pay attention to students' background and learning style, in order to find out the best strategies for the specific group.

Munro (1985) underlined the importance of being aware of the attitudes to which students are exposed: "The general attitude of the staff and the faculty toward research, their interest, or lack of it, are far more important in shaping the students' attitudes than all the research classes and seminars that one might design'' (p. 368). Referring to these elements, much attention has to be paid to involving the clinical staff in research projects, not only to change their attitude and enhance their skills in order to let them become a research resource, but also influence positively students' attitudes toward research. In fact, often clinical staff are asked to cooperate in some ways in nursing education, but less has been done to help them develop their competence to do so. Continuing education programs have to offer this opportunity. However, they are mostly oriented toward clinical skills. In the future it has been recommended that researchers involve clinical staff to achieve the following goals: (a) their cooperation in data collection; (b) the introduction of research findings in clinical practice; and (c) improved teaching to students of research.

According to Harrison, Lowery, and Bailey (1991), few researchers have evaluated empirically the effects of research courses on students' attitudes toward or knowledge about research. Most of the articles described teaching experiences directed toward undergraduate students. In fact, most difficulties have been described in enhancing baccalaureate students' attitudes. A few authors described courses to Master's students.

Even if most of the studies are not research-based, they can offer interesting starting points to develop research projects. Research on teaching approaches and methods is not easy to develop, for many reasons. First, the research can take a long time. Secondly, comparison groups are not easy to find and control. Third, even introducing quasi-experimental designs, many variables are difficult to control. A short description of strategies introduced and methods utilized in teaching research is reported below.

Baccalaureate Students

Overfield and Duffy (1984) reported reviews on teaching approaches of 11 studies from 1967 to 1980: studies of undergraduate research: contents, instrumentation and findings (five studies from 1966 to 1981); and studies of nursing education and implementation of research (three studies between 1978 and 1981). Beck (1988) listed strategies for teaching nursing research published by the *Western Journal of Nursing Research* in the years 1979 to 1986. An overview of teaching strategies is presented. Even if all the reported studies are helpful to generate ideas, many have internal consistency problems, therefore, their results can be questionable.

Shell and Crain (1992) reported a repeated experience to introduce research. They invited undergraduates of five local baccalaureate programs to attend a Research Day. A call for posters was sent to the larger nursing community and the response was good. The themes of the first 4 years were the following: overview of nursing research; nursing diagnosis: implications for research; nursing research in clinical practice; and development and diversity: back to basics. The half-day meetings were attended by three to four hundred people. A questionnaire submitted to participants and returned by almost half confirmed interest by the attendees. Such an experience seems to the author valuable as a first general introduction into research; as Shell and Crain write, "an opportunity for socialization concerning research for the total undergraduate student body at one time" (p. 20). Referring to Italian experiences of introduction to nursing research (CEREF 1992, 1993), conferences are most effective when attendees already have a research background and if students' own research projects are presented.

Munro (1985) suggested the use of clinical conferences to help students see where research is needed to answer questions and solve dilemmas. Champion (1988) reported a successful strategy following a pervasive approach. It included incorporation of positive statements about research into each lecture and lectures given with enthusiasm; conscious attempts to demonstrate the value of research to professional practice; role modeling incorporated into the research course; projects of the instructor and other colleagues included as examples; and clinical nurses currently conducting research serving as guest speakers. The positive results were assessed by an attitude assessment scale.

Rajacich, Kane & Foster (1991) reported a 10-student experience doing research in a community setting. They identified the "lack of membership growth of a senior retiree club" as a researchable problem. Subsequently they developed a research project. A survey was conducted for a 3-month period. The project enabled students to witness the applicability and efficacy of research.

Molloy and Isaak (1989) also provided students with a community research experience. Twenty-eight students in medicine, nursing, and dental medicine had the opportunity to participate in a research project during the summer clinical training. Students participated in the design of the data collection tools and served as data collectors. Some entered the data on the computer at the side and assisted with the categorization of the data. Part of the value of the learning experience was the discussion and the sharing of insights among students from different schools. Students appreciated the opportunity to participate in a research process firsthand in a "real world" setting.

Gueldner et al. (1993) involved students as research assistants in an outdoor 12-week walking intervention involving ambulatory nursing home residents at multiple sites. Students' research role was to assist in the implementation of the prescribed treatment conditions, administration of questionnaires, and even coding and entering data into the computer. In another project they were requested to recruit and test individual subjects for the development of an instrument. Results that were described with enthusiasm by the students were an increase in research skills, command of a new sophisticated language, and an appreciation of the importance of communication. Moreover, along the way more and more responsible behaviors in accomplishment of research tasks were noted. Collins, Corder-Mabe, Greenberg, & Crowder (1992) offered a similar opportunity to students in maternal-child nursing. Ludmann (1981b) included students in the collection of data for a community health assessment project developed by faculty. Attention was given to use this work as a teaching strategy, having students to really integrate the assigned task with other learning activities.

A "short answer progressive assignments" methodology was used throughout the semester by Laschinger, Docherty, & Dennis et al. (1992). Students chose a topic of personal interest and carried this study through the various phases of the research process. Feedback and positive reinforcement ware provided continuously by faculty. Short mid-term tests and a final multiple choice exam were added to the evaluation produced through the assignments. Positive results were obtained from the assignments, the exam, and the students' judgements of the usefulness of the strategy.

Fowles (1992) suggested a poster presentation as a strategy for evaluating students. Students had to arrange a poster using an article's content. The assumption was that students must be able to comprehend and evaluate the components of a research report to prepare a poster.

An experience to promote qualitative research application among students was reported by Harrison, Hubbard, and Lane (1987). During the clinical practicum carried out during their last semester of their senior year, two students were involved in confirming the findings of a previous study. They observed, kept a written log describing their impressions and clinical experience each day, and discussed the research with professionals in order to elicit their perceptions. Results showed the development of interest toward research and the willingness to utilize research in practice. Another experience of teaching qualitative research methods was reported by Bull (1992). In addition to class work, every student was involved in interviewing older adults about their health. They also worked in small teams to refine an interview guide, share literature, decide on specific criteria for sample selection, code and analyze the data, and prepare oral and written reports of their findings. All the students but one enjoyed the experience and asserted that they had developed a better attitude toward research. Beck (1988) introduced the students to research, proposing to them to "try on" the image of nurse researcher. They conducted a phenomenological study of a caring nurse/client experience from the client's perspective. They went through a process of categorization.

Critiquing skills were the core of the course implemented by Van Bree (1981). Students were required to write a critique of an article and prepare to lead a discussion based on it. In addition, they had to carry out a small project in groups of two or three. A question that could be answered by a descriptive study was chosen.

An experience to promote students' understanding of the theory-research-practice concept and the use of explicit nursing models as frameworks for nursing research questions was realized by Laschinger et al. (1992). Students were asked to evaluate the appropriateness of the use of nursing models in research articles. Moreover, they had to search the literature for appropriate nursing conceptual frameworks to fit in a research question identified by themselves. The authors' assumption was that nursing research questions should be placed within nursing conceptual frameworks.

Harris (1985) introduced computer-assisted instruction (CAI) lessons in a research course. Four tentative answers were allowed students before giving the correct one. Students were provided with lesson text material, questions, and students' answers to take home. Statistics were kept each time a student took a lesson. Reis and Wright (1992) described a nursing research methods course designed around the use of three types of computer software: tutorials, patient education, and statistics. The course was scheduled for six 2-hour computer labs and the same amount of time for lessons and discussions.

Anderson (1992) introduced students to the concepts of research utilization, projecting a list of validated innovations on a transparency. Students were asked to indicate their awareness of them and if they had implemented them. Results of the survey were discussed among the students and with faculty. The approach could be further developed and perhaps become more effective if students would have to find out a list of innovations, having a chance to look up the literature.

Organizational aspects connected to carry out a research project, such as communication in the research group and with other involved subjects, have been described in a students' experience by Schare (1977). Even if they contribute to a project's success, often they were not adequately considered in teaching research methodology. In the same article an interesting aspect was underlined, and unfortunately not sufficiently supported by research, by the authors or by others: the opportunity to allow students to make errors in planning in order to learn.

Results were assessed on attitudes toward the importance of nursing research, increase in confidence in being able to do nursing research, increase in interest in conducting research, personal comfort, importance of computer literacy, necessity of a computer background to use computers, and acceptance of statistical software in nursing research. No results on knowledge were reported.

A quasi-experimental study was conducted by Harrison et al. (1991) using both critiquing and proposal development. Students critiqued articles and completed objective examinations and small group work. Findings showed that students developed positive attitudes. Even if at the end of the research course there was an increase in knowledge, no significance was shown between the pretest and the final test at the end of the nursing program. As a consequence, the authors raised questions about the effectiveness of the traditional course in pursuing ANA (1981) aims. Based on the studies' results, they changed the teaching, introducing identification of more researchable problems and applications of research findings.

Pennebaker (1991) assessed through a survey costs and benefits of the use of collaboration among students in carrying out research projects. Her results confirming a preference of the students to select collaboration rather than working alone are supported by Poletti et al. (1993). Pennebaker underlines an important point: "Students are not only challenged with the complexity and difficulty of clinically oriented research, but also with the knowledge that nursing research often requires cooperation if findings are to be meaningful and translated into practice" (p. 107).

Master's Students

Selby and Tuttle (1985, 1988) utilized successfully the guided design strategy. Firlit et al. (1986) asked students working in small groups to identify a patient care problem, search the literature for studies of nursing interventions related to the problem, critique these studies, and develop a protocol according with the studies that meet the scientific criteria. The protocol "synthesizes the research base related to the nursing intervention, or innovation, and describes the research design and methodology prescribed to implement and evaluate the innovation in a clinical trial" (p. 107). Afterwards, the methodology used in a clinical trial of the innovation and the plan for analyzing and interpreting data were added. The author underlined the use of a group approach as more realistic in a clinical setting. A compound strategy was developed by Beal (1989) using modeling as a central pivot. Warner and Tenney (1985) tested the relative effectiveness of lecture and computer-assisted instruction (CAI) using two groups of students in a research course. No significant difference was shown. However, the researchers underlined a need for using both the methods in a compound way.

Post-basic education

A survey was conducted by the teachers of 38 centers where a general intensive care course for registered nurses in England was carried out (Stanley, 1989). Twelve teachers filled in the submitted questionnaire. The strategies used in courses to teach research were class-based and used lectures and discussions, a project development or a research critique, literature searches, care plans, case studies, or essays based on research findings. A connected survey by the same author through a questionnaire submitted to 12 course members showed that the most appreciated part in the course was the project, through the data collection and the analysis of the findings.

Continuing education

Swanson, Albright, Steirn, Schaffner, & Costa (1992) described a multi-branched approach to develop interest and knowledge among clinical nurses. They proposed short courses (2 to 6 hours) on specific points of methodology, such as "introduction to writing and publication for nurses;" meetings with authors of clinical research projects, who could describe their own work and results; a nurse-to-nurse consultation having a specialist consulting through reporting the last results of research referred to a specific problem, even personally or by a written response; and a focus-oriented distribution of published material to wards.

An important feature most of the authors introduced (Harrison et al., 1987; Van Bree, 1981) was to offer students the opportunity to present their work to peers, faculty professionals, and so on. The opportunity motivated the students, and gave them an impulse to better understand the topic, produce in a publishable manner, and learn to communicate. Beal's students (1989) practiced for their presentations at a research symposium using a videotape. Posters have been one of the most popular way of presentation and many authors introduced it in their courses (Firlit et al., 1986; Fowles, 1992). Kirkpatrick and Martin (1991) provided specific information regarding poster preparation. Van Bree (1981) posted a report of student projects on a research bulletin board near the student lounge. Fawdry and Temple (1989) provided important suggestions concerning the content to be taught to teach research communication.

There are many didactic methods used for teaching research. A few of them are considered here referring to their use for the specific purpose. A general analysis of their effectiveness is presented in the chapter describing teaching methods research.

Methods used for teaching research are the lecture; discussion; games; role playing; consequential task (Laschinger et al., 1992); field trips; computer-assisted instruction; projects; assigned readings; and writing and poster preparation and presentation. Brand (1991) introduced a game, a crossword puzzle, to teach students basic research terms, capturing the imagination while reinforcing content. It was used for both group and individual efforts. Levin (1988) used role playing to help students to prepare to utilize research in the clinical practice applying communication skills and focus on possible obstacles. Data collection simulations were introduced by Ludmann (1981b) such as telephone or face-to-face interviews with classmates or responding to and then analyzing a questionnaire given to class. Kirchhoff (1991) described the use of field trips, the first to an individual who was using research in formulation of unit or institutional policies, and the other was to participate in a journal club. One major goal of the activity was to provide students with role models so that they could visualize themselves participating in research.

Results were positive, as research was seen by students as a plausible activity, both for staff nurses in clinical setting and for themselves. Reading research reports was the strategy introduced by Ludmann (1981a). Students worked in groups of three, read and discussed reports, and then described the study to the rest of the class. This method can help students to have an overview of the research methodology. This is very important, because if they have a long way to go before the conclusion, they do not have a clear idea of the goals; therefore it is difficult to arise and keep motivation toward the task. Sorrell (1988) reported a three-step experience. Students had to produce: (1) in-class writing to personalize each step of the research process; (2) one-page abstracts to promote skills in summarizing complex information; (3) one-page critiques to encourage analytical thinking about the research process. The author described learning as occurring by personalizing the content through writing in class, putting themselves into the mind of the researcher before writing a summary, and standing outside the research process as a critiquer. Nerone (1987) suggested asking students to write for publication and encouraging them to write a query letter. To accomplish this task students have to investigate the most likely journals to publish the article, and they have to pay attention to have followed the research process to have the article accepted.

FURTHER DEVELOPMENT

Much more attention has to be given to teaching research in the nursing schools of all levels. As a consequence, research has to be increased. Main issues are the following: (a) To develop comparison research to assess the effectiveness of different approaches, and use of different didactic methods; (b) follow-up studies; (c) needs assessment of the required research competencies by nurses in all positions; and (d) studies on transferability of research skills from research area to other professional areas. In conclusion, teaching research has to move from only graduate students to also undergraduates and professionals; from class to include clinical and community settings; from research methodology to applied methodology and statistics; from lessons to include the use of active methods; and from exclusively research-oriented to popular in content. As a consequence, in the years to come literature on teaching nursing research is expected to move from experience reports to more research-based studies; from few articles to many articles; from description of teaching to include description of outcomes methods; and from American authors to international authors. Worldwide cooperation is needed to assess cultural differences, evaluate contexts' impact, and enrich research opportunities. As a consequence, knowledge in nursing's disciplinary domain will be enhanced.

REFERENCES

Abel, E., & Sherman, J. J. (1991). Use of national data sets to teach graduate students research skills. *Western Journal of Nursing Research, 13,* 795–797.

American Nurses' Association [ANA] Commission on Nursing Research. (1981). *Guidelines for the investigative functions of nurses.* Kansas City: Author.

Anderson, E. T. (1992). Student awareness of research findings. *Nurse Educator, 17,* 12–14.

Beal, J. A. (1989). Strategies for teaching nursing research: The use of modeling in teaching nursing research on the graduate level. *Western Journal of Nursing Research, 11,* 247–250.

Beck, C. T. (1988). Strategies for teaching nursing research: Review of "Strategies for teaching nursing research," 1979–1986. *Western Journal of Nursing Research, 10,* 222–225.

Brand, K. (1991). Strategies for teaching nursing research: A crossword puzzle can teach research terms. *Western Journal of Nursing Research, 13,* 278–283.

Bull, M. J. (1992). Using qualitative methods in teaching undergraduate students research. *Nursing and health care, 13,* 378–381.

Bzdek, V. M., & Ganong, L. H. (1986). Teaching the research process through participatory learning. *Nurse Educator, 11,* 24–28.

Center of Research and Education. (1992). *Teaching research methodology and statistics in nursing school.* Proceedings of the first regional conference. Venice, Italy: Regione del Veneto.

Center of Research and Education. (1993). Teaching research methodology and statistics in the nursing school. *ISIS News, 8,* 2–23.

Champion, V. (1988). Research teaching strategies. *Nurse Educator, 13,* 5.

Collins, B. A., Corder-Mabe, J., Greenberg, E., & Crowder, D. S. (1992). Strategies for teaching nursing research: Incorporating a research study into undergraduate clinical. *Western Journal of Nursing Research, 148,* 677–680.

Fawdry, M. K., & Temple, A. (1989). Strategies for teaching nursing research: Even in research, the medium is the message. *Western Journal of Nursing Research, 148,* 677–680.

Firlit, S. L., Kemp, M. G., & Walsh, M. (1986). Strategies for teaching nursing research: Preparing master's students to develop clinical trials. *Western Journal of Nursing Research, 8,* 106–109.

Fowles, E. R. (1992). Poster presentations as a strategy for evaluating nursing students in a research course. *Journal of Nursing Education, 31,* 287.

Gueldner, S., Clayton, G. M., Bramlett, M. H., & Boettcher, J. (1993). The undergraduate student as research assistant. Promoting scientific inquiry. *Nurse Educator, 18,* 18–21.

Harris, S. L. (1985). Development of computer assisted instruction. Lessons for teaching nursing research. *Computers in nursing, 4,* 140–141.

Harrison, L. L., Hubbard, L., & Lane, J. (1987). Confirmation of qualitative research findings in the clinical setting: A strategy to promote research application among baccalaureate nursing students. *Journal of Nursing Education, 26,* 208–210.

Harrison, L. L., Lowery, B., & Bailey, P. (1991). Changes in nursing students' knowledge about and attitudes toward research following an undergraduate research course. *Journal of Advanced Nursing, 16*, 807–812.

Kirchhoff, K. T. (1991). The use of field trips in teaching nursing research. *Journal of Nursing Education, 30*, 89–90.

Kirkpatrick, H., & Martin, M. (1991). Strategies for teaching nursing research: Communicating nursing research through poster presentation. *Western Journal of Nursing Research, 13*, 145–148.

Kovacs, A. R. (1974). Research for the undergraduate student in nursing. *The Journal of Nursing Education, 13*, 31–36.

Laschinger, H. K., Docherty, S., & Dennis, C. (1992). Helping students use nursing models to guide research. *Nurse Educator, 17*, 36–38.

Lee, K. (1988). Meta-analysis: A third alternative for student research experience. *Nurse Educator, 13*, 30–33.

Levin, R. F. (1988). Strategies for teaching nursing research: Role-play to simulate application of research findings. *Western Journal of Nursing Research, 10*, 782–785.

Ludmann, R. (1981a). Strategies for teaching nursing research: Experiential learning in data collection. *Western Journal of Nursing Research, 3*, 249–251.

Ludmann, R. (1981b). Strategies for teaching nursing research: First class sessions are crucial to success. *Western Journal of Nursing Research, 3*, 116–117.

Molloy, C., & Isaak, M. (1989). Baccalaureate students learn research and teamwork in a community setting. *Journal of Nursing Education, 28*, 36–38.

Munro, B. (1985). Promoting enthusiasm for research among undergraduate students. *Journal of Nursing Education, 24*, 368–371.

Nerone, B. J. (1987). Preparing students to write for publication. *Nurse Educator, 12*, 34–35.

Overfield, T., & Duffy, M. E. (1984). Research on teaching research in the baccalaureate nursing curriculum. *Journal of Advanced Nursing, 9*, 189–196.

Pennebaker, D. F. (1991). Teaching nursing research through collaboration: Costs and benefits. *Journal of Nursing Education, 30*, 102–108.

Poletti, P., & Vian, F. (1992). Experimental teaching in methodology of research and statistics in nursing schools. In *Voyage into the future through nursing research: Proceedings of the International Research Conference*. Indianapolis, IN: Sigma Theta Tau International (Pub.), 148.

Poletti, P., Vian, F., & Vittadello, F. (1993). An approach to teaching research methodology and statistics in the nursing school. An experiment in Veneto. *La Formazione del Medico, 7*(4), 18–22.

Rajacich, D., Kane, D., & Foster, M. (1991). A practical approach to teaching nursing research. *Nursing Forum, 26*, 17–21.

Reis, J., & Wright, S. (1992). Computers and undergraduate nursing research: A pilot study. *Journal of Nursing Education, 31*, 237–238.

Selby, M. L., & Tuttle, D. M. (1985). Teaching nursing research by guided design: A pilot study. *Journal of Nursing Education, 24*, 250–252.

Selby, M. L., & Tuttle, D. M. (1988). Guided design: Evaluation of a model for teaching nursing research. *Journal of Nursing Education, 27*, 303–308.

Schare, B. (1977). An undergraduate research experience. *Nursing Outlook, 25*, 178–180.

Sorrell, J. (1988). Strategies for teaching nursing research: Writing to learn nursing research. *Western Journal of Nursing Research, 10*, 511–514.

Spector, N. C., & Bleeks, S. L. (1980). Strategies to improve students' attitudes to research. *Nursing Outlook, 18*, 300–304.

Stanley, H. F. (1989). A study of the teaching of nursing research using the project method to post-basic registered nurses on ENB Course 100 (General intensive care nursing for RGN). *Intensive Care Nursing, 5*, 171–174.

Swanson, J. M., Albright, J., Steirn, C. Schaffner, A., & Costa, L. (1992). Strategies for teaching nursing research: Program efforts for creating a research environment in a clinical setting. *Western Journal of Nursing Research, 14*, 241–245.

Van Bree, N. (1985). Preparing faculty to teach nursing research. *Journal of Nursing Education, 24*, 84–86.

Van Bree, N. (1981). Undergraduate research. *Nursing Outlook, 29*, 39–41.

Warner, S., & Tenney, J. W. (1985). Strategies for teaching nursing research: A test of computer-assisted instruction in teaching nursing research. *Western Journal of Nursing Research, 7*, 132–134.

Woodtli, A. O. (1990). Strategies for teaching nursing research: The honors research project. *Western Journal of Nursing Research, 12*, 566–570.

CHAPTER 9

Integration of Clinical and Theoretical Teaching

Margaret F. Alexander, RGN, SCM, RNT, BSC, PhD, FRCN

WHY INTEGRATE CLINICAL AND THEORETICAL TEACHING?

> *"Then," said a teacher, "Speak to us of Teaching."*
> *And he said:*
> *"No man (or woman) can reveal to you aught but that which already lies half asleep in the dawning of your knowledge. ...*
> *"If he (the teacher) is indeed wise he does not bid you enter the house of his wisdom, but rather leads you to the threshold of your own mind."*
>
> **(Gibran, 1926, p. 26)**

Good nursing is such a mixture of the very simple and of the extremely complex. Good nursing, which we can all recognize when we see it but are only recently beginning to articulate, is a totality, a whole, which is very much more than the sum of the parts. The wise teacher of the art and science of nursing does not endeavor to reduce the complexity of nursing to the banal, the simple, only a series of discrete tasks, to be learned by rote; nor does he/she espouse, or encourage his/her students to search for one all-encompassing model or theory of nursing. Rather, using his/her own knowledge and experience of practice, and the insights gained from reading, research, and from patients and others who write eloquently of their personal experience of the reality of nursing care, he/she endeavors to lead his/her students to the threshold of their minds, to encourage in them an enquiring, analytical way of thinking about nursing which will never leave them. He/She teaches about his/her concept of nursing, a holistic concept, in which nursing practice and theory, clinical teaching, and theoretical teaching are so much part of the same cloth, the same pattern, as to seem indivisible. To relate to nursing what Gibran (1926) describes so beautifully, in relation to other professions, the nurse teacher, and the practicing nurse who teaches, can speak only of *their* understanding of nursing; they cannot *give* that understanding to the student. The dawning of understanding, of new knowledge, the actual integration and synthesis of the clinical and theoretical teaching, of practice with theory, must take place within the student's own mind (Alexander, 1983; Halliburton, 1976). Their teachers, if they believe in the necessity to integrate clinical and theoretical teaching, can of course help by designing the curriculum, and their teaching, in such a way as to encourage that synthesis from the very beginning of the education of entrants to nursing, and throughout the continuing education programs they design for qualified nurses.

Listen to a true story of practice, shared with her classmates and her teachers, by one of our first-year students. The students had been studying, in class, what it meant to be "a person"—the concept of "personhood." What a difficult concept for a class composed mainly of young people aged around 18 years of age to grasp. "But we know what being a person means, why do we have to learn this abstract stuff? What has this to do with real nursing?" They struggled with this amongst other theoretical teaching—and longed to be in the wards with the patients. Then . . . (and this was one student's story):

> I was caring for an old gentleman who was lying in bed. He told me he wanted to pass urine. I asked him if he wanted a urinal, or to get up to the commode or to go to the toilets at the foot of the ward. He wanted to go to the toilet and so I helped him to get up, to put on his dressing gown and walked with him, holding on to my arm, down to the toilet. At the door, I asked if he thought he could manage on his own, but he said no, he didn't think he was steady enough and wanted me to come in with him. I did—and closed the door, standing beside him and steadying him. Suddenly, the door burst open and one of the other nurses on the ward said—"Come on, Mary, I've been looking for you—it's time you went to your coffee break. If you're going to get it you'll have to go now."—and she left. Suddenly, I understood what it means to be a person, to have dignity, to have rights. Had that nurse herself been using the toilet, she would have been absolutely horrified to have her privacy interrupted—yet it was as if the old gentleman did not exist—yet alone exist as a person, a fellow human being. Now I understood, now I could see how that so-called theoretical knowledge was so important to my practice of caring, my practice of nursing. (First year student, 1992/93 BA/BA (Honours) Nursing, Glasgow Caledonia University)

The integration, the synthesis, had occurred in the head of the student— her way of thinking was undergoing a process of change; she stood at the threshold of new learning. Her teacher had a wisdom, an understanding of nursing, which the student could not fully reach at this early stage. She could not enter the teacher's "house of wisdom," but what a giant leap forward she took in her own mind, in her personal understanding of the connections between practice and theory in these few moments . . . and how the theory was informed—and transformed—by the student's experience of this single episode of nursing, or, as Christensen (1993) would say, of working in partnership with this patient.

THE DEBATE

Let us look at "our nursing," as Nightingale (cited in Skeet, 1980) puts it. The raison d'etre for all nurse education, and indeed nurse education research, is ultimately the provision of the best possible standard of patient–client care. Education is a means towards that end. It sounds simple. Why, then, is there considerable debate about the best means towards that agreed end? And why has the debate gone on for so long? Will there ever be one right answer—and therefore an end to the debate?

In this chapter it is proposed that there will not—nor ought there to be—only one right answer for nursing education; that debate is healthy and is essential because there is no static end-point. Individual, community, and national needs for nursing are not static. They change and develop. Our knowledge about nursing likewise changes and develops, particularly now that it is very gradually becoming more informed by research. Let us examine just some of the challenges and issues which surround one element of the nurse education debate—the integration of clinical and theoretical teaching, which is viewed as synonymous with the integration of practice and theory.

DEFINITIONS

Clinical teaching, is defined as teaching which takes place *mainly*, but not exclusively, in the world of practice, be that in hospital or in the primary health care setting, i.e., the community. *Theoretical teaching* is defined as that which takes place *mainly* in the university or other academic institution where nursing programs are offered, i.e., in the classroom. However, there is not always, nor should there be, the clear-cut difference which is normally inferred when these two concepts are written about or discussed. Indeed, part of the dichotomy which is and has long been perceived between the two arises from the tendency to think of these two essential elements of nurse education as taking place in two different places, and being conducted by two different groups of professional nurses, i.e., the academics, the teachers or lecturers, and the practitioners. Of course, this is mainly the case, but how would one describe the increasing use, by the educator in the classroom, of vivid accounts of the lived experience of ill health as told by patients or clients, of the portrayal of caring in the visual arts, of paradigm cases or stories of practice as illustrated at the start of this paper? Is that no clinical teaching, teaching which is focused on the reality of practice? How would one describe the increasing use of technology in the Nursing Skills Laboratory, to focus not just on the technical accuracy of the performance of psychomotor skills such as the conduct of aseptic technique, but on the verbal and nonverbal communication which accompanies such a procedure, which might be performed on a fellow student, or on an actor, portraying a patient? Is that not also a form of clinical teaching? How would one describe the qualified practicing nurse's application of knowledge of the physiological theories of homeostasis, of acid-base balance, or of the psychological theories of learning when caring for a patient and also acting as a role model for a student nurse, and subsequently explaining to the student the rationale for nursing actions? Is that not theoretical teaching? While we accept that *in the main*, clinical teaching and theoretical teaching take place in two different settings, and *in the main* these two elements are conducted by qualified, experienced nurses whose post-registration education has taken two different routes, the edges are blurred, there are no firm boundaries around each, and indeed the interplay is the key factor. This view will contribute to a positive debate about the way forward for nurse education and nurse education research.

THE NATURE OF NURSING: IMPERATIVES FOR INTEGRATING CLINICAL AND THEORETICAL TEACHING

All that now follows is based upon what may seem an obvious assumption, but, if one delves deep, is not necessarily a reality in all parts of the world; and that is that education is essential for the world's nurses; that the availability of a well-educated nursing workforce is essential to the health of the individual, the community, and the nation and that the rightful work of the nurse is the promotion of health and the prevention of disease, as well as the care of those who are ill. This is the position taken clearly by the World Health Organization in its policy documents and in its description of the Health for All Nursing Series (WHO, 1991, 1991a). But the provision of a health service is an extremely expensive outlay for governments. The provision of a nursing service represents a very large part of that expenditure, and throughout the world, we are being faced with politicians who query not just how many qualified nurses are needed, but what is their contribution in terms of outcomes, what kind of skill mix is necessary in order to obtain efficient, cost-effective outcomes, and what education is necessary for the qualified nurses and their helpers. In the discussion of the integration of clinical and theoretical teaching for the entrants to nursing, and for the qualified nursing workforce it is important to bear this in mind.

It is the author's belief that the nature of nursing creates an imperative for integrating the clinical and theoretical aspects. Moore (1990, p. 825) states: "Nursing, as a discipline, not only encompasses knowledge, but how that knowledge is translated into practice." and "He who knows theory but not the practice does not know the whole theory." (Perkins, 1965, cited in Moore, 1990, p. 826).

The main reason why clinical and theoretical teaching should be integrated is simply because, when we conceptualize nursing, what we remember, what we think about, are our patients or clients, and our interactions with them. The patients, because *we* come from all over the world, will represent humanity across our world. The experience of nursing them, for each one of us, will be uniquely ours; its practice, a blend of the art and science of nursing.

William Blake, an English poet, (1757–1829) said "For art and science cannot exist but in minutely organized particulars." Nursing is about putting together into a coherent whole all of these tiny "particulars" or details of caring, wherever that care is delivered, whether in a high technology, acute care hospital, in a health center, or in a patient or client's own home.

Thus, nurse education is about putting together into a coherent whole the theoretical, equated here with the pure science and technical rationality as described by Schon (1983, 1987), and the artistic or aesthetic. Education for nursing should place an equal value on both. But history is against us, for centuries there has been a tension between the scientific and the artistic. Schon (1987, p. 30) sketches in the history of the Positivist position, i.e., the "dominant view of professional knowledge as the application of scientific theory and technique to the instrumental problems of practice. . . . According to the Positivist epistemology of practice, craft and artistry had no lasting place in rigorous practical knowledge" (Schon, 1987, p. 34). Practice was of a lower order than theory . . . and the taint of that hierarchy remains with us today and is at the root of many of the problems of the integration of the clinical with the theoretical. Schon (1983, p. 42) graphically depicts the dilemma of "rigor or relevance" in the practice disciplines, of which nursing is one. He contrasts what he terms "the high hard ground" of rigorous professional knowledge, where problems are amenable to solutions by the application of rules and practitioners can make effective use of research-based theory and technique, with the "swampy lowland" where situations and problems are confusing, may defy objective technical-rational solutions, but are often of the greatest human concern. His metaphors reinforce the notion of a hierarchy of knowledge, with the scientific and the theoretical of more importance than the practice or the clinical.

Is it any wonder that nursing students and their teachers alike tend to compartmentalize and elevate the science, and see as of a lesser order in the hierarchy of knowledge, the art, which is equated with practice?

Schon, whose work has been, and continues to be very influential in nursing, suggested that we turn the question of professional knowledge on its head and search for "an epistemology of practice" implicit in the artistic, intuitive processes which some practitioners bring to situations of uncertainty, uniqueness, and value conflict. In other words, that it is our tacit knowledge, our "knowing-in-action," derived from our "reflection-in-action" (Schon, 1983, p. 50) which is central to the art by which expert nurses deal with the unique, context-dependent work of nursing. Meerabeau (1992), in a thorough exploration of tacit nursing knowledge, considers that practitioners' knowledge is an important and largely untapped resource which should be the subject of more research—perhaps in the form of cooperative inquiry between researcher and practitioner. This author proposes that this cooperative inquiry might occur also between researcher and teacher.

Powell (1989) used Schon's work as the theoretical background to her small but in-depth study of eight practicing nurses and their use of reflection-in-action in their everyday work. As a very experienced nurse and educator, her research interest was in finding out how nurses learn from experience, if indeed they do so, given that professional practice is essentially individual (Powell, 1989) and thus defies routinization or rigidity. Her results indicated a certain amount of reflection-in-action on the part of these experienced nurses, but this was at a relatively superficial level. They tended to separate theory from practice and were unable to maximize the potential of learning from their nursing work. Powell, however, later went on to create a very innovative curriculum for a post-registration honors degree program in nursing in which practice, and reflection-on-practice, was central. Students of this degree, all experienced nurses, working in practice or in education, explore the value of theoretical knowledge to practice, but above all, learn how practice can inform and generate theory. This curriculum certainly leads these students, many of them experts in their field, to the threshold of their minds, and the dawning of new knowledge. There is clear evidence in their coursework that this is so and also in their ability to change practice—and in their commitment to lead new entrants to the profession to that valuing of practice, so essential to the breaking down of the barriers between the clinical and the theoretical.

From the author's experience of teaching such mature students in her own Department, it is clear that they readily see the relevance of certain theories to their clinical practice and are hungry to learn more, but it takes them longer to understand that practice can in fact inform theory.

In the University of Western Sydney at Macarthur in Australia, Andersen (1991) has, together with colleagues, built an entire nursing curriculum around her belief that practice should drive theory, which in turn should inform practice. Andersen's project arose, more than 18 years ago, from a challenge she was given to provide a research basis for a tertiary-level nurse education program. The paradigm which drove Andersen's curriculum project (Gray & Pratt, 1991, p. 122) highlights the interrelationship between practice, reflection on practice, and theory, a spiral illustrating that the integral whole is more than the sum of the parts. From day one, students in this program study "real" practice scenarios, and are required actively to seek out knowledge, from diverse disciplines as well as from nursing, in order to aid their understanding of what is happening in a particular patient care scenario, and to decide what nursing actions might be appropriate. The apparent simplicity of the model disguises the long process of enquiry and reflection which led Andersen to her conceptualization of the nature of nursing as a dynamic, interactive, and goal-oriented activity, a discipline in its own right, in which inquiry processes guide interventions which are chosen in order to enable people, or groups of people to engage in activities of daily living, to maintain health and/or to cope with disease, *in collaboration with* their nurses. (Andersen, 1991).

Making the voice of the consumer heard and influential in the care he or she receives is the focus of the "Nursing Partnership," as conceptualized by Christensen (1993), also a nurse and educator from the Antipodes, in her fresh new way of examining the "mutual work" which occurs during what Christensen describes as a "shared journey" when "a nurse offers learned expertise to a person who is passing through a health-related experience." Christensen also adds a temporal dimension to the nurse/patient encounter and explicitly comments on the artistry: "Nursing is continually shaping and reshaping in response to the complexities inherent in the present and ongoing circumstances of each patient's passage. This process has been likened to that of an artist at work." (Christensen, 1993, p. 29). So, again, we hear of the situation-dependent dimension in the expert nurse's work with patients which Benner (1984) illustrates, i.e., "They (the expert nurses) know how to function in the face of unpredictable situations and adjust their plans to the contingencies of the situation" (p. 115). Christensen's Nursing Partnership model rings true because it is derived directly from practice. She describes her model in use in practice, but interestingly, also in education, where the passage of the student reflects both a giving and a receiving, a partnership, composed of her own work, the work of the educator, the work of the role model practicing nurse, and the work of the patient. In harmony with the philosophy of partnership, Christensen never prescribes, but offers the model she has created, and which she is continually revisiting and developing in collaboration with colleagues, to all of us, to use, experiment with and modify, so that it works for us, and our students, patients or clients. Nothing is finite in the Nursing Partnership model; just a clear message that *nursing matters*, practice is paramount.

Just because practice is so situation-dependent, it follows that no one theory, model, or approach will suffice. Rather, theoretical pluralism is required, as Moore (1990) amongst others advocates; but also required is that valuing of the knowledge generated from practice and a recognition that such knowledge can and should influence the development of nursing theories.

Goldstein (1986), writing in relation to social work, challenges the assumption that effective or "good" practice must be rooted in an established theoretical foundation and that without this, the quality of practice suffers. He argues that the gap is not between theory and practice, but between theoretician and practitioner, that the reality is known in a way which is different from that prescribed by theorists; that theories are reductionist myths and that we must consider other modes of understanding which have a more common-sense and humanistic nature and in which the voice of the recipient of care is influential. In this way, Goldstein's work is in harmony with that of many of the authors cited above, the essence of which is that nursing is a practice discipline, and that practice is paramount. It seems, therefore, that it is axiomatic that those who teach nursing, must also practice nursing, and so be able to integrate both the clinical and theoretical aspects of the whole.

THE ROLE OF THE NURSE TEACHER IN INTEGRATING CLINICAL AND THEORETICAL TEACHING

It is important also to concentrate on the role and contribution of the nurse teacher, while not in any way diminishing the critical contribution of the education given by the practicing nurse, whether as a role model as he/she goes about his/her daily work of nursing, or as a designated mentor or preceptor. The reason for concentrating on the nurse teacher is because, at this time in the United Kingdom, we are facing challenges in relation to the role of the nurse teacher which are directly related to the issue of the integration of practice and theory, or clinical and theoretical teaching. Although there are some differences between countries, it is safe to assume that many of these challenges are similar in other countries in Europe and indeed globally, to a greater or lesser extent, and to review them briefly will inform the debate, as well as suggesting questions for future research. We can all learn from each other's experiences and perhaps particularly nurse educators from the countries of Central and Eastern Europe, who are building up their nurse education programs anew, or who are in the process of reorienting them away from a medical model towards a nursing and primary health care model, can learn from these descriptions.

More than 8 years ago, in the UK, statutory bodies were set up, under government legislation, to govern the preparation required for nursing and to maintain a register of qualified nurses, intended to safeguard the patient by ensuring appropriate standards (Baly, 1973). Some years later, a key report (Lancet Commission on Nursing, 1932) suggested that ward sisters be relieved of some of their duties to enable them to spend more time teaching nurses in what the report stated unequivocally was a craft. Over the years, student nurses gradually became entitled to periods of time out from practice, to be spent in the classroom, learning the theoretical aspects of their discipline of nursing. Much of this "training," as opposed to education, was rote learning of nursing procedures to be carried out "on" passive patients, a far cry from the partnership Christensen (1993) described, and the remainder tended to be lectures from doctors about anatomy and the pathophysiology of various disorders. The focus of nurse training was clearly on disease, not health; and on hospital, not community or primary health care settings. The fact that, for the vast majority of patients, their period of hospitalization was a relatively brief, though perhaps very influential, episode in their lives, and that of their families, seemed seldom to be considered.

Gradually, not only was the time spent in theoretical instruction increased, but material from what are now seen as essential supporting disciplines, such as biological sciences, sociology, political science, psychology, and communication studies, was integrated into the curriculum, and the students' nursing clinical experience was extended and broadened. Unfortunately, as the syllabus grew in breadth, nurse teachers were expected to be masters of all trades and found they were required to teach everything. For many, their efforts to keep abreast of a relatively elementary syllabus in these supporting subjects, resulted in their expert nursing knowledge, their clinical expertise, becoming gradually eroded.

In the 1950s, in the UK, two grades of nurse teacher were created, each with formal teaching qualifications, the Registered Nurse Teacher and the Clinical Teacher. This was done because it was becoming very obvious that the qualified teachers of that time were seldom, if ever, in the clinical areas, helping the students to integrate their theoretical preparation with their practice, and because the ward sisters and staff nurses, although committed to and conducting a certain amount of supervision and teaching of student nurses, were unable to devote sufficient time to this. The creation of the two grades was done with the best of intentions. Clinical teachers had a very specific remit, to bridge the gap between theory and practice. It is interesting to note that the formal qualifications required in order to teach the complexities of the practice of nursing in the clinical areas were of a lesser order than those required if one was to teach in the classrooms! (Alexander, 1983; Vaughan, 1990).

Over the years, what had seemed a logical solution to the integration of clinical and theoretical teaching patently did not work out as intended. Many registered nurse teachers became classroom teachers only, ever more entrenched in the ivory tower of the classroom and divorced from the reality of practice. The clinical teacher, as a "guest" in the clinical areas, without any overall responsibility for patient care, therefore with little or no influence on standards of practice became frustrated and felt something of a "second-class citizen"—"belonging" neither in the university or college, nor in the wards and other areas of clinical practice.

Various initiatives took place, in an effort to bring theory and practice closer together. Different forms of joint appointment, between education and service, were developed and evaluated (King Edward's Hospital Fund for London, 1984). The concept of the lecturer/practitioner was developed particularly in Oxford, and Lathlean (1992) reported an ethnographic study of this innovation. These lecturer/practitioners have authority and responsibility for practice, setting standards and preparing staff and the environment to create the optimum climate for the delivery of a high standard of patient care and for student learning. In addition, lecturer/practitioners share with others the responsibilities for the development and delivery of the nursing modules in the students' educational programs, thus being in an ideal position to integrate the clinical and theoretical teaching (Champion, 1992). It is proving to be a difficult and taxing role, highly rewarding for some, but too stressful for others. There should be many useful lessons to be learned from the results of this, the first major evaluation of the lecturer/practitioners in action.

Taking a different tack, work being done at McMaster University in Canada highlights a successful collaboration between educators, clinicians, and managers. There they have designed three types of university and service appointments (Kirkpatrick, Byrne, Martin, & Roth et al., 1991). The evaluation of this initiative indicated advantages to both the hospital and the university in a strengthening of links, an increased mutual respect between practitioners and educators and, at the center, enriched learning opportunities not just for the students, but for those who teach them.

The author's doctoral research was an educational experiment designed to facilitate the closer integration of theory and practice. The participants were the teachers, and control and experimental groups of student nurses, in 6 of the then 19 colleges of nursing and midwifery in Scotland (Alexander, 1982; 1983). In this research, the two grades of nurse teacher had identical roles, i.e., they taught in both classroom and in the clinical areas; they taught both theory and practice. Students received the "theory" of the care, in this case of patients suffering from disorders of the gastrointestinal system, in the classroom. Then, still during their study time, they went to the clinical areas to nurse patients with the disorders about which they had just been learning. The students were supernumerary to the staffing of the wards, a situation which at the time was not the norm. They returned from their experience of supervised practice to reflect upon the individualized, total patient care which they had given, and shared this reflection with their group and the teachers who had supervised them. The results of this study showed that not only, over time, were the students in the experimental group able to retain more of the nursing knowledge they had gained than were their counterparts in the control group, but their valuing of this method of integrated teaching, and their insights into nursing, were both discerning and positive. Their teachers, although in some cases frankly acknowledging a feeling of stress in returning to the clinical areas, were also positive about this approach to the teaching of nursing.

However, in spite of all these various initiatives, the registered nurse teacher in the UK tends to remain within the classroom and away from the reality of practice.

In the late 1980s, all four countries of the UK discontinued the two distinct forms of preparation and the two grades of nurse teacher, returning to one grade only, that of the registered nurse teacher. At the point when the UK entered upon the biggest change in our nurse education system almost since its inception, i.e., the new preparation for practice entitled Project 2000 (United Kingdom Central Council for Nursing, Midwifery and Health Visiting 1986), we did so with only one grade of nurse teacher, who was expected to integrate clinical and theoretical teaching.

Much has changed. Nurse teachers are better educated, more and more toward the degree and higher degree level. There is a slowly growing acceptance that they should be experts in research-based nursing, and that this is what they should teach, allowing the experts in the contributing disciplines to teach other subjects. The nurse teacher can then explore with her students, be they entrants to nursing or qualified nurses continuing their education, how to apply and adapt, where relevant, the theoretical concepts, and indeed the research from these disciplines, to nursing.

But the debate still rages. A search of the last two years of the major research-based UK nursing journal and the UK journal which focuses specifically on nurse education has revealed a considerable number of articles on the role of the nurse teacher. Research by Crotty and Butterworth (1992) and Clifford (1993), amongst others, indicates that this is still a very varied role, but with little or no teaching being done in the patient care areas. Crotty (1993) wrote, following a Delphi survey of 25 colleges of nursing in England, and in-depth interviewing of a small group of 12 teachers from 6 colleges, that:

> None . . . currently undertake any clinical teaching which involves giving care to a patient with a student. This is contrary to what was anticipated in Project 2000 programmes, as it was expected that the teacher would supervise and teach patient care. The interviewees did not feel that teaching by giving "hands-on care" was part of their role. They felt that this was the role of the qualified staff in the clinical areas. (p. 463)

This is a view genuinely held by quite a number of nurse teachers, not just in the UK. A study in Norway found that teachers there had made the decision that it is the role of the practicing nurse to supervise and teach the students in the clinical areas, and that it is not their role as teachers (Crotty, 1992).

The author's view is that the nurse teacher *must* be there, in the reality of practice, or on the swampy lowlands, as Schon (1983) puts it. He/she must be with the student who is experiencing that practice, sharing the learning and caring. It is not necessary, indeed it would be unrealistic and counterproductive, for the nurse teacher to be there all the time that the student is in practice. But unless the teacher of nursing is regularly immersed in the practice of nursing, he/she cannot maintain his/her clinical expertise, and cannot share the students' "lived experience" of practice, cannot empathize with the student and the patient of today. A teacher of nursing who is not practicing nursing is bound to lose credibility with his/her colleagues in practice and with his/her students. His/her "bank" of nursing knowledge, no doubt credible in her early days as an teacher, becomes less and less so as time goes on and he/she is inevitably more and more divorced from the context-dependent, complicated reality of practice. In regularly touching base with practice, the teacher's own wisdom and understanding is growing and deepening, so that he/she is in a position to lead the student towards his/her own growing understanding. The learning opportunities are endless, individual and often, never-to-be-forgotten experiences. What is being taught to and hopefully learned by the student, when teacher, student and patient are together in a partnership in giving and receiving nursing care, in a *way of thinking* about nursing; not just a series of tasks, performed on a passive patient by a detached professional.

The following is an example from the author's own research—an example never to be forgotten. It occurred when a student in the experimental group attended the ward, with her teacher, to undertake nursing care. The patient, cachectic, exhausted, and terminally ill, was lying silently in bed, his large and eloquent eyes looking at us. Sister had asked the student nurse to bathe him. The Kardex notes were available to the teacher and student, but were being used by other nurses, so they both, at this point, went first to meet the patient and then to prepare their equipment. The student, only 6 months into her pre-registration education program, said to her teacher, almost bitterly, "What can I learn—he cannot talk to me—there's nothing I can do except wash him. It's not fair, I'm here to learn." It is only natural that, at this very early stage in her knowledge and experience of nursing, this student nurse was quite simply seeing only the superficial, not the totality of the situation. What fundamental nursing values *might* she have formed had she not been with her teacher at that time? What a wealth of opportunity was open to the wise and skilled teacher—not just to teach and help the student learn about the essential techniques in the giving of the physical care, the so-called "basic" nursing, but to take the student on a journey, to try to enable her to be open to learning a whole way of being in relation to what nursing, what skilled caring is about. This individual man, at this point in time in his life, isolated from family and familiar environments and suffering from a terminal illness, presented the nurse teacher with so many intangibles which defy rigid routine, the high hard ground of professional knowledge, but which cry out for the sensitivity, the artistry of the process of giving that nursing care. The happier outcome to this episode was of a dawning of knowledge in this student nurse, just a beginning of wisdom, of a new way of thinking about practice, of being sensitive, in a holistic way, to the lived experience of one patient whose every communication, voiceless as it was, was about being so helpless and so alone, in the midst of the exhausting bustle which surrounded him, of endless interruptions as nurses came and went, changing his dressings, adjusting his intravenous fluids, aspirating his nasogastric tube.

Two major reports which include proposals for the education and subsequent practice of nurse teachers in the UK have been commissioned. The consultation period for the *Report on Standards for Post-Registration Education* from our main Statutory Body for Nursing, the United Kingdom Central Council, (UKCC 1993) has just closed. This report has a very welcome emphasis on practice and proposes a new framework of continuing education to prepare Specialist Practitioners and Advanced Practitioners for practice beyond the level achieved following initial registration as a nurse. In order to become a nurse teacher in the future, the Report proposes that the practitioner must be a graduate, hold an advanced nursing qualification, have relevant and up-to-date clinical experience and the ability to teach effectively. Staff in the author's department, in preparing a response to the consultation document, were wholeheartedly in agreement with this proposal. We feel work must begin soon to provide the requisite courses and also the practice opportunities for nurse teachers to regain their clinical expertise. We also pointed out that there are considerable funding, logistical, and accommodation implications in this proposal which must be addressed and discussed with the providers of health care services. We look forward to the publication of the results of the consultation exercise.

Our professional organization, the Royal College of Nursing, has just issued a discussion document which proposes a more radical solution to the problem of the preparation of teachers of nurses. They recognized that intensive staff development will be needed to enable teachers to reestablish their own practice competence and to consider ways to develop their role in the practice setting. They rejected the continuation of the present role, holding on to tradition, as they express it. They also rejected the trend for some nurse teachers to prepare themselves to degree level in subjects other than nursing, predicting that, in the long run, this will lead to them being seen as "cuckoos in other birds' nests", (Royal College of Nursing [RCN],

1993). They strongly advocated practice-oriented teacher preparation and forecasted that the nurse teacher of the future will be first and foremost a practitioner whose degree is in nursing. He/she will be someone who regularly switches, on a 2- to 5-year cycle, between practice and teaching, management of nursing services and teaching, or research and teaching. In other words, their radical scenario is that nurse teaching will no longer be a job for life!

Part of the reason for these current proposals is the findings from some of the research into nurse education, which are providing more and more evidence of the divorce of the teacher of nursing from the practice of nursing and of the lack of integration of clinical and theoretical teaching.

THE RESOURCE IMPLICATIONS OF A TRUE INTEGRATION OF CLINICAL AND THEORETICAL TEACHING

One very important factor which is relevant to the recreation and development of this dual role for nurse teachers too often remains unspoken; that is the funding of nursing programs. The funding of nursing departments (or faculties) in the university or higher education sector in the UK, and perhaps in other countries too, has not ever been sufficient to provide a staffing resource which can enable effective delivery of meaningful clinical teaching as well as theoretical teaching and opportunities to update practice. Currently, where academic staff are regularly supervising students in the clinical and primary health care settings, and where such integration of the clinical and theoretical is being done well, highly committed staff tend to be overstretched and work very long hours. Not only is this not acceptable practice, but their workload makes it extremely difficult for them to conduct research and publish, both essential scholarly activities for academic staff, and on which they, and the departments and universities for which they work, are judged. The staffing resource, i.e., the staff-student ratio, also influences the ability to deliver a student-centered curriculum. In order to encourage the student to link theory and practice, there must be space in the curriculum for reflection-in-action, which can only be delivered by using labor-intensive teaching and learning strategies, and labor-intensive clinical assessment strategies. The battle for adequate funding is one that departments of nursing must fight continually.

THE PROCESSES OF TEACHING, LEARNING AND ASSESSMENT WHICH PROMOTE INTEGRATION OF THEORY AND PRACTICE

Not only should the structure of the curriculum be such as to juxtapose relevant theoretical and clinical experiences for the students, but teaching, learning, and assessment should be seen, as in Christensen's model (1993) as a partnership between student and teacher. Within the author's own department, and particularly in the preregistration nursing degree program, teaching and learning is regarded as a two-way process between students and staff. The perception is that learning occurs when material is seen to be relevant and when concept networking can take place. For this to occur, whenever possible the learning should be practice-generated. In our program, too, students generate part of their own syllabus by deciding, on the basis of their clinical or other learning experiences, what is relevant knowledge for them to seek. Prompts are supplied by teachers, who also ensure that professional competencies as laid down by the statutory body are met. Having identified the theme or problem they wish to investigate, the students undertake a broad-based literature review eliciting the help of academic and clinical staff as appropriate. The theme is then written up by the student, along with other evidence, and gradually a portfolio of relevant knowledge is assembled (Glasgow Caledonian University (GCU), 1992). Lecturers (faculty) in the preregistration program all share responsibilities for clinical supervision and regularly supervise students in their practice placements. Course work and assignments in nursing are focused on the integration of theory with practice, as is the clinical assessment profile. The intention behind this program is that the student is at the center of the learning process, engaged in an eclectic approach to learning, and emerged as a competent and knowledgeable practitioner. Similarly, with the programs for qualified experienced nurses, staff seek to encourage this independent, questioning approach to research-based practice.

How do we view our teaching? Fox (1983) found, when he asked teachers "what do you mean by teaching," that four basic conceptions emerged:

> There was the "transfer theory," which treats knowledge as a commodity to be transferred from one vessel to another. There was the "shaping theory" . . . molding students to a predetermined pattern . . . the "traveling theory" . . . (where there are) hills to be climbed for better viewpoints, with the teacher as . . . an expert guide, and finally there was the "growing theory" which focuses more attention on the intellectual and emotional development of the student. (Fox, p. 151)

What we are trying to do is to help our students to grow, in their knowledge and understanding of the art and science of nursing. We hope that one of the outcomes of this approach will be practitioners who value practice and the theory which informs and is informed by that practice, and who respond creatively to the climate of change in care delivery.

WHAT OF THE FUTURE—WHAT IS THE WAY FORWARD?

The way forward can only be via continuing debate and via research, research on the relationships between nurse education and practice, and theory and practice; research into how professionals think in action and into the outcomes of that reflective, creative thinking process in terms of benefit to the patient; and rigorous evaluation of examples of good practice in nurse education. Gradually, as more nurses and teachers gain an understanding of the research process, such research should be a collaborative effort between teachers, practitioners, and researchers, because nurse education is in essence a collaborative effort among all three groups. There is also a need for more multidisciplinary research, because many of the issues in nurse education are mirrored in education for members of other practice disciplines.

Pirsig (1974) writes:

> "What's new?" is an interesting and broadening eternal question but one which, if pursued exclusively, results only in an endless parade of trivia and fashion, the silt of tomorrow. I would like, instead, to be concerned with the question of 'what is best?'—a question which cuts deeply rather than broadly, a question whose answer tends to move the silt downstream. (p. 7)

Dialogue, mutual trust, and a growing understanding between teachers, practitioners, managers, and researchers are essential if we are to seek and find the best ways of integrating theory and practice in nurse education, and if we are to continue to refine and adjust that education, so as to maximize the potential of the nurse's contribution to the health and the nursing care of the people of our various countries. We must do it together—and I am sure that we can.

REFERENCES

Alexander, M. F. (1982). Integrating theory and practice in nursing, Part I and Part II. *Nursing Times, 78*, 17–18.

Alexander, M. F. (1983). Mapping the terrain of the discipline. In G. Gray & R. Pratt, (Eds.), *Towards a discipline of nursing* (pp. 95–123). London: Churchill Livingstone.

Baly, M. E. (1973). Nursing and social change. London: Heinemann.

Benner, P. (1984). From novice to expert: Excellence and power in clinical nursing practice. New York: Addison-Wesley.

Carter, G. B. (1939). A new deal for nurses. London: V. Gollancz.

Champion, R. (1992). Professional collaboration: The lecturer practitioner role. In H. Bines and D. Watson, (Eds.), *Developing professional education* (pp. 113–118). London: Open University Press.

Christensen, J. (1993). Nursing partnership: A model for nursing practice. Longman Group.

Clifford, C. (1993). The clinical role of the nurse teacher in the United Kingdom. *Journal of Advanced Nursing, 18*, 281–289.

Crotty, M. (1992). The activities of nurse teachers in the Diaconia College, Oslo, Norway. *Senior Nurse 12*, 33–37.

Crotty, M. (1993). Clinical role activities of nurse teachers in Project 2000 programmes. *Journal of Advanced Nursing 18*, 460–464.

Crotty, M., & Butterworth, T. (1992). The emerging role of the nurse teacher in Project 2000 programmes in England: A literature review. *Journal of Advanced Nursing, 17*, 1377–1387.

Fox, D. (1983). Theories of teaching. *Studies in Higher Education, 8*, 151–163.

Gibran, K. (1926). *The prophet* (1991 edn.) London: Pan Books.

Glasgow Caledonian University. (1992). *BA/BA (Honours) Nursing Studies Definitive course document*. Glasgow: Glasgow Caledonian University Health and Nursing Studies Department.

Goldstein, H. (1986). Toward the integration of theory and practice: A humanistic approach. *Social Work, 31*, 352–357.

Gray & Pratt. (1991). *Towards a discipline of nursing*. London: Churchill Livingstone.

Halliburton, J. C. (1976). *Internal evaluation of an experimental datum curriculum in a diploma school of nursing*. Unpublished EdD. thesis, Boston University School of Education.

King Edward's Hospital Fund for London. (1984). Joint clinical-teaching appointments in nursing. London: King's Fund.

Kirkpatrick, H., Byrne, C., Martin, M.-L., & Roth, M. L. (1991). A collaborative model for the clinical education of baccalaureate nursing students. *Journal of Advanced Nursing, 16*, 101–107.

Lancet. (1932). The report of the Lancet Commission on Nursing. London: *The Lancet*.

Lathlean, J. (1992). The contribution of lecturer practitioners to theory and practice in nursing. *Journal of Clinical Nursing, 1*, 237–242.

Meerabeau, L. (1992). Tacit nursing knowledge: An untapped resource or a methodological headache? *Journal of Advanced Nursing, 17*, 108–112.

Moore, S. (1990). Thoughts on the discipline of nursing as we approach the year 2000. *Journal of Advanced Nursing, 15*, 825–828.

Persig, R. M. (1974). *Zen and the art of motor cycle maintenance*. Corgi Books.

Powell, J. H. (1989). The reflective practitioner in nursing. *Journal of Advanced Nursing, 14*, 824–832.

Revans, R. W. (1978). *The ABC of action learning*. Manchester: Altrincham.

Royal College of Nursing. (1993). *Teaching in a different world: An RCN discussion document*. London: Royal College of Nursing.

Schon, D. (1983). *The reflective practitioner*. New York: Basic Books.

Schon, D. (1987). *Educating the reflective practitioner*. New York: Jossey-Bass.

Skeet, M. (1980). *Notes on nursing: The science and the art*. Edinburgh: Churchill Livingstone.

United Kindgom Central Council for Nursing, Midwifery and Health Visiting. (1986). *Project 2000: A new preparation for practice*. London: Author.

United Kingdom Central Council for Nursing, Midwifery and Health Visiting. (1993). *The Council's Proposed Standards for post-registration education*. London: Author.

Vaughan, B. (1990). Knowing that and knowing how: The role of the lecturer practitioner. In B. Kershaw & J. Salvage (Eds.), *Models for nursing* (pp. 103–113). Scutari Press.

World Health Organization. (1991a). *Health for all nursing series*, No. 1–7. Copenhagen: Author.

World Health Organization. (1991b). Reviewing and reorienting the basic nursing curriculum Health for All Nursing Series (No. 4). Copenhagen: Author.

CHAPTER 10

Teaching of Clinical Judgment in the Czech Republic

Marta Stankova, PhD

C linical judgment plays a key role in the quality of nursing. The teaching of clinical judgment in the course of preparation of nurses for their profession is different in different countries because it depends largely on the system of education at nursing schools, on the curricula, and particularly on the organization and methodological guidance of practical or clinical training in clinics.

The level of clinical judgment depends on many factors, that can be divided into two groups: *Pedagogical factors*, comprising the curriculum, the method of teaching clinical judgment in both theory and practice, and the system of organization of practical training—at a clinic, the nursing staff's involvement in teaching at a clinical department; and *psychosocial factors*, including the age and social maturity of the students, the ability to link theoretical clinical knowledge and experience in the process of decisionmaking, the time when they are taught clinical judgment, and the level of their professional decision making in a particular clinical situation.

It is important to first attend to some specifics of teaching in clinical practice in relation to the development of students' skills in clinical judgment.

In European nursing education, there exist two different systems of students' clinical practice which considerably influence the ways of teaching clinical judgment. In most of the western countries students apply their theoretical and practical skills and knowledge of clinical judgment directly in nursing care and are supervised by the experienced staff nurses. In contrast to this system, in some countries of Central and Eastern Europe the students are supervised during practical training predominantly by the nurse teachers.

Both systems have some positives and some negatives which influence also the teaching methods of clinical judgment. Post-Socialist nursing is characterized especially by task-centered nursing care in which the nurse is oriented to carry out doctors' orders. Clinical judgment of patients and the identification of patients' needs at the current hospital ward plays a secondary role. Consequently, students supervised only by staff nurses are not directed to the evaluation of the clinical status of patients, but to the instrumental nursing skills.

This is the reason why there is a preference for the system in which nurse-teachers try to develop students' skills in clinical judgment, not only during the theoretical lessons at school but also during the clinical practice of the hospital ward.

During the last 2 years in the Czech Republic nurse educators have organized a number of courses for nurse-teachers with the assistance of foreign lecturers oriented to the teaching of nursing process and clinical judgment in clinical practice.

The following is a presentation of some results of the study which was performed at the three nursing schools and which documents some positive effect of the study. Selected results of the experiment have demonstrated that modernization of practical training, stressing activation teaching methods, can develop students' skills directed at clinical judgment. In addition, students learn to solve both clinical and human problems of patients, while simultaneously training in manual skills is of secondary significance.

METHOD

The experimental education was directed at the following aims:

- Full and effective utilization of time in practical lessons;
- Systematic long-term development of professional perceptiveness, observation, and communication skills of students;
- The students' inner identification with the model of nursing care, and their instruction in the active application of nursing's general characteristics to a particular clinical situation with regard to the patient's disease and biopsychosocial-specific features; and
- Training of professional nursing skills to be performed in close connection with practicing nurses from the very beginning of the practical training at the clinical facility.

The experimental education program was based on the following principles. First of all, a set of activation teaching methods elaborated in accordance with nursing school conditions were used. The method of individualized care was the most typical of the methods. In addition to the usual tasks, students assumed more intensive care of a particular patient. They were solving the patient's problems more deeply and in greater detail, getting to know him/her and treating him/her in an active way. They were learning to identify themselves with patient status and trying to solve problems actively. The relationship between nurse and patient was formed in a natural and spontaneous way.

The second principle was to intensify the home preparation for practical lessons. This homework involved dealing with special problems set beforehand to be solved later at the course. The homework also included students' written reports on their patients, the so-called case reports. Each case report contained the patient's characteristics, evaluation of his/her needs and clinical status, and a proposal of an active care plan. In the following days the student attempted to carry out the plan.

The third basic principle of the experimental teaching/learning process was based on the strong involvement of the members of clinical staff in practical lessons. The staff nurse participated in students' performance, demonstrating to them the correct procedure. The nurse-teacher was concentrating on activities concerning the clinical judgment and individual nursing care. Nurses also took part in theoretical lessons, where individual patients were discussed in greater detail. They also assisted the teacher in assessing the students' skills and behavior regularly at the end of the lesson.

The experimental model was tested on students from the second, third, and fourth courses at three Nursing Schools. The lessons took place in clinical units of medical departments in hospitals. The results of the three experimental groups were compared with those of three control groups where the practical training took place in a traditional way.

Three methods were used to assess the experiment:

- Observation of the students treating the patients;
- Analysis of the written case reports; and
- Evaluation of the students' behavior in problem model situations.

RESULTS

In all experimental groups the students' activity was considerably higher than in control groups by an average of 30%. In the analysis of the individual criteria studied, the greatest difference was found in preventing the complications of immobilization syndrome (mobility activation, respiratory exercises, constipation prevention, pressure sore prevention, etc.). These are the most important activities coming from a good level of clinical judgment of patients. A great difference was also found in the care of mental comfort of patients, which is influenced by clinical judgment and communication skills.

The second assessment method analyzed the written case reports elaborated in the experimental groups and the thesis written by the control groups. The students' ability to understand the clinical problems of individual patients and their proposal for an appropriate treatment were assessed. The nursing case reports of the experimental groups were successful in as many as 80% of the cases, but only in 50% of the control groups. The biological problems of the patients were solved similarly in both groups of students. The reports of the experimental group were more complex, including also the psychological and social areas. Students were able to elaborate the information by providing a broader and more complex specification of the patient's clinical problems from the nursing point of view.

To establish the degree of independence and responsibility, the students' behavior in a model situation was assessed. The patients, who had been instructed in advance, mentioned some alarming defects in front of the student (e.g., dyspnea, acute pain). The next steps of the students were observed— how students would treat the information obtained, whom they would pass it over to, and how they would manage the situation. In the quantitative evaluation, four behavioral elements were assessed: the mere realization, dealing with the piece of information in greater detail, materialization, and presentation to responsible staff.

In experimental groups, more than 90% of students noticed the information, while in the control groups, only 75% did so. In the latter groups, 25% of students remained ''deaf'' to the patients' information. This fact is somewhat startling. Though the absolute results of the experimental groups were considerably better than those of the control groups in other criteria as well, it has been proven that the lower class the students attend, the less likely they are to be engaged in the situation and the less their sense of responsibility. Essentially, they will remain unconcerned.

The investigators also were interested in the person being referred to in case of students' spontaneous help. The students of the experimental groups passed the information on more frequently (70%, in comparison with 43%). The range of competent persons was also wider, including the teacher, nurse, and physician. One-half of the students passed the information over to two persons. The conclusion can be drawn that the active involvement of the clinical department staff in practical lessons increases the students' sense of appurtenance to the team, which is extremely important from the point of view of staff relationships.

The general evaluation of the experimental teaching/learning process proves the experiment to be successful. The parameters of professional activity in clinical judgment were nearly 30% higher. Activation methods produced higher cognitive of students, improving the frequency and quality of clinical judgment of patients and appropriate nursing care. The cooperation of students, teachers, and nurses resulted in development of good professional relationships and higher professional responsibility. The best results were achieved in the fourth course, where emotionally and socially mature students showed a responsible attitude to their patients and were able to make better use of all their professional knowledge and experience in systematic clinical judgment. The level of the manual skills was not impaired in the experiment.

CONCLUSION

The proposed model aiming at the development of clinical judgment skills is effective, feasible, dependable, and performable in practical terms. It provides good preconditions for the development of professional activities of future nurses. However, it is necessary to continue developing these basic skills even after the nurse has started his/her professional practice, i.e., within the health team. In that case, such humanized and highly professional nursing becomes a common model both for new students and for nurses starting their professional practice.

CHAPTER 11

Issues in Developing a New Model for Nursing Education

Majda Slajmer–Japelj, RN, Soc.

W hen building a new study program in nursing in countries where the traditional "medical models" of nursing have been used before, we have to consider many issues. The main topic in the past was illness; during their programs of study, the students concentrated on illness and were enchanted by the dynamics of the treatment of disease. Health promotion and prevention was a minor part in the program. Health was too abstract for the students. For this reason most of the young graduates were interested in work in large clinical institutions. The medical model, which did not give the possibility for independent professional thinking among nurses, influenced students and future graduates. The main and most important part of a subject was the medical part, as in surgery, internal medicine, pediatrics, e.g., and nursing was just an appendix to the medical information. The medicoclinical component was taught by physicians and there was no discussion possible, and no questions were expected from student nurses. The contents were given as axiom. They had to be accepted and followed. This expected behavior in the classroom was later transferred into practice, and therefore the hierarchy of health professions within the health system did not give nursing any chance for the independent decisions so necessary for the development and effectiveness of a profession. Practical exercises in the hospital institutions allowed very few deviations from the existing routine of nursing services. The exception was community nursing, where the individual work of students, under the supervision of community nurses, enabled them to think and to work independently. Using the medical model, most nursing schools were not able to develop a professional and scientific language for the profession. The medical language was the only professional language. The words "anamnesis" and "diagnosis" were sacred and reserved only for physicians.

The schools and boarding houses for nursing students were isolated from other students; therefore, nurses had difficulties integrating into different strata of the society, and they did not build their interpersonal contacts with the students of other professions who would support their work after graduating. In addition, the new concept of understanding a successful national health system that includes multisectoral cooperation for all who are involved in health care was not stressed.

The deficits in past education of nurses demonstrate the importance of both a proper conceptual framework and an organizational framework of a program. The first priority for better quality is teacher preparation in nursing. Further, to be able to meet the needs of the population, nurses have to be mostly interested in health; therefore, their educational programs have to start with the development of a healthy individual, family and community. They have to study pathology, which should be accompanied with the measures of primary and secondary prevention. They have to learn how they will help to bring an individual, a family, and a community to the highest possible state of health, or will help them to live independently with the consequences of illness or trauma through the cooperation in health, social, and perhaps also professional rehabilitation. Also the school has to be independent in professional decisions, but integrated into the academic society of the country.

The quick change from a traditional model into the modern and very adaptable integrated model of work is not possible overnight. There are many handicaps, such as:

- existing university legislation, which is sometimes very rigid;
- unclear financial regulations;
- the conservative mentality of teachers who want their own small area without discussion of other views;
- the classic examination system, assessing only the memorization and retention capacities of the students and not asking for critical judgment;
- the strong differences that still exist between hospital and extramural nursing; and
- the attitude of caring only for individuals, and not for the health of society.

When we want to start a nursing program with a new philosophy, we have to also decide what type of a school we shall build. If the profession is already strong and independent, then we can propose the model of a "University for Health Sciences" with some common parts of the program for all health professions. If this is not the case, we should start with a separate nursing school, but should organize, together with other educational schools for health professions, some common programs; for instance, the study of the health problems in a village as a case study, the reorganization of a health institution, or similar cases. Even the complex health treatment of individual clients/patients could be a very useful educational team experience.

The whole educational concept has to have a firm thread: from wellness to illness and back to wellness; from simple to complex problems, from the individual to the community, from conception till death.

The responsibility of the educational institutions is high, "Because nursing is what nurses are and nurses are what the schools make them. . (Woodtli).

REFERENCES

Woodtli, A. (1993, September). *Women's health*. Presentation at the International Conference.

PART III

Issues Important to Nurse Educators Worldwide

CHAPTER 12

The Process of Professional Identification

Kornelia K. Helembai, RN, PhD

T he most important task of professional nursing education is to help students acquire the knowledge and skills that will enable them to perform nursing tasks independently. In preparation for professional practice, however, it is not enough to master knowledge needed to perform nursing tasks successfully; students also have to understand the reciprocal role expectations of the nurse/patient relationship. Through understanding the role expectations of both partners in the relationship, students learn the norms of professional behavior (Zakar, 1988). These professional behavioral norms which are derived from societal expectations are not entirely dependent on specific personality traits, but the process of the development of students' professional identity and role-related behaviors are influenced by individual students' personality characteristics.

NURSE/PATIENT ROLE RELATIONSHIPS

The nurse/patient relationship is regulated by the rights and duties inherent in the nurse's and the patient's roles. Role partners expect from each other certain behaviors in advance. It is expected that behavior meet predetermined reciprocal role requirements, i.e., that the patient's rights become the nurse's duties (Csaszar, 1980). The effectiveness and outcome of the nurse/patient relationship is thus influenced by each partner's mutual role expectation and their abilities to modify their own behavior. In the nurse/patient relationship, it is the professional nurse who is expected to reduce tensions and solve problems within that relationship by using professional knowledge and skills in order to make optimal decisions in the interest of the patient's health. Regulation of internal tensions and the manifestation of tolerance is expected of the nurse for successful decisionmaking.

Faulty interpretation of expected role behaviors can lead to disturbances in interactions between nurses and patients that create a sensation of uncertainty and tension. This tension in turn affects decisionmaking and, eventually, the development of career identification.

Nurses need to regulate their own behaviors and decisionmaking during the course of their professional activities. This necessitates that each nurse control and direct her/his behavior. The ability to do this, however, is based on several factors within the nurse and within the environment. Such factors are the psychovegetative and emotional balancing, the degree of personal development and maturity of the nurse, and such factors in the environment as the pressure of time to select and make optimal decisions, the patient's previous experiences in similar situations, and the ability of both patient and nurse to make dynamic adaptations.

THE PROCESS OF CAREER IDENTIFICATION

Two major phases of professional career identification process have been identified: the *anticipated identification* and the *real career identification* processes. Each phase consists of two minor processes, the sub- and preidentification processes leading to anticipated career identification during the students' formal education. The primary identification and the secondary identification processes lead to the real career identification, which occurs during the early years of nurses' careers (Helembai, 1989). Career identification begins with the clarification of individual role expectations and their mutual compatibility, resulting in subidentification. The acquisition of role components potentially suitable for independent practice with clarification of the patient's (role partner's expectations leads to the nursing students' preidentification and results in the anticipated career identification.

During the primary identification phase, the new graduate explores the compatibility of role expectations with the expectations of and compliance with the changing demands of patients (role partners). Secondary identification occurs later in the professional nurse's career, with actual compliance with the expectations of patients, when their changing needs and demands have been fulfilled. The last step in the process through which real career identification is attained occurs with the realization of individual variations and the development and internalization of a pervasive nature of the professional role.

Variables Affecting the Process of Professional Career Identification

In order to assess the levels of career identification of students and practicing nurses, variables affecting the process were studied using several psychological tests. Findings of interest are the result of longitudinal studies conducted by the author (Helembai, 1989). Two major areas were explored: (a) specific conditions of self-regulation and (b) the success of self-regulation in a relationship. The following variables were studied to explore the relevance of self-regulation to professional career identification: (a) characteristics of information processing; (b) the formation of social behavior; and (c) indexes of psychovegetative and emotional balancing.

Under the general category of self-regulation in a partnership the variables included were: (a) the characteristics of relationship formation, (b) the solution of conflict situations; and (c) the traits affecting regulation of internal tensions. Correlations between these variables were not found to be significant; however, they appear to influence professional career identification. Results of the study, although not generalizable, point to the need to coordinate students' intrapersonal development, their interpersonal skills, and the knowledge needed for professional practice.

The center of professional nursing practice is the nurse/patient relationship. In this relationship the nurse becomes the "work-instrument." If this premise is accepted, then students must know and understand the self, and learn self-regulation in professional relationships as they must master other professional knowledge. This can only be achieved through a theoretically sound educational plan.

REFERENCES

Csaszar, G. (1980). *Psychosomatic medicine*. Budapest, Hungary: Akedemiai Kiado.

Helembai, K. (1989). *Where the object of the work is the human being*. Budapest, Hungary: Pedagogiai Szemle.

Zakar, A. (1988). *Theories of choice of career*. Budapest, Hungary: Tankonyvkiado.

CHAPTER 13

The Importance of Including Ethics in Nursing Education

Zeinab Loutfi, RN, PhD

E thics, as defined by Fordham (1992), is the science of morals, the branch of philosophy which is concerned with human character and conduct. Nursing ethics is primarily concerned with the application of the science of morals to what is considered right or wrong in the conduct of human relationships between nurses and all those people with whom they come into contact in their professional capacity. Much of the time, thinking about ethical issues is implicit rather than explicit, and behavior is motivated by an amalgam of ethics, etiquette, and pragmatism, tempered by awareness of legal constraints. According to Harris (1968), "The source of moral obligation is the greater good, and nursing has its origins in this moral obligation" (p. 117). Churchill (1977), in his discussion of ethical issues facing nurses, stated that "Ethics is the free, rational assessment of courses of actions in relation to principles, rules, conduct" and that "Critical self-examination is the heart of ethics" (p. 873).

WHY NURSING ETHICS?

Through advances in medical technology, the opportunities for intervening in patients' destinies by restoring heartbeats, respiration, kidney function, hearts themselves, and possibly optimum genetic composition are many. The future promises even more ways of controlling vital functions and altering body parts. Nurses are part of these interventions. At the primary level of prevention and care, patients and families look to their nurses for information, advice, and support when facing difficult decisions of this nature. At the secondary level of curative care, nurses are actively involved in monitoring and sustaining treatment modalities, such as life support systems. At a societal level, nurses are expected to be actively involved in policy formulation within the health organization both in professional societies and in legislative bodies.

Thus, nursing is an integral part of the health care delivery system. The practitioner of nursing is in continuous contact with the patient and the fam-

115

ily. This position offers unique privileges and responsibilities. Nurses are the nearest to the patient's most intimate fears, hopes, and regrets. By word and deed, the nurse manifests to the family a sense of caring and of fundamental human dignity.

Nurses, according to Bandman and Bandman (1985) "strive to meet universal human needs for care in illness and for the prevention of disease. Nurses seek to conserve that which is of value to every individual - the optimum functioning of all body systems and of the whole as an integrated unit" (p. 2). Above all, nursing is a human health service that has the quality of mercy. Nursing's practice, as described by Patridge (1978), is concerned with humans and is humanizing (p. 360). A central concern of nursing practice is to enhance the personhood and the humanity of all involved in care.

Indeed, the nursing of the well and sick is identified with doing "good." But why is nursing good? It is good because there is not an act of nursing that does not aim at what is identified as the "good" in common sense terms. But good intent is not enough, since knowledge or ignorance of alternatives is a cause of good or harm. Reasons for choosing one alternative over another, or refusing treatment altogether, need to be critically examined in relation to other possibilities. Moreover, nurses wish not to impose their treatment choices on other persons whose autonomy is to be supported. The nurse's beliefs concerning the good life may differ from those of the patient. It is precisely this difference that needs to be acknowledged and respected as a mark of personhood and separateness. Knowledge, therefore, of the ethical views that support reasons for one choice over another are indispensable to the nurse in daily practice and in everyday life. Thus, the function of nursing ethics is to guide the activity of nursing on behalf of the good.

CONSIDERING THE ALTERNATIVES

Many values must be considered by nursing professionals when making ethical decisions. According to Ney (1991), the first and most important are the patients' values, such as the care they should receive while hospitalized. In addition, patients may have certain needs and expectations because of their disease processes, their experience, and their personal value systems. Likewise, the value system of families may influence ethical decisionmaking; patient and family may or may not share the same values. An ethical dilemma may be created by disagreement between the patient and family about the course of treatment.

The values of the various members of the health care team also impact ethical decisions. These team members may include physicians, social workers, respiratory therapists, and other nursing professionals. Each discipline and individual has a perspective and a unique contribution to ethical patient care.

Structural values are also of concern when resolving ethical dilemmas. The structural values most often implicated include institutional issues, e.g., hospital policy, procedures, or protocol, and legal issues.

Lastly, societal values play a role in ethical problem-solving. Some of the values societies may hold include use of all available technology to preserve life versus limited resources allocations; death as a part of life versus life at all costs; or respect for the aged versus emphasis on youth and vitality.

With all these values influencing nursing professionals, ethical problem-solving may seem an insurmountable task. Resources must be available to support and guide nursing professionals through the ethical dilemmas.

NURSES' ETHICS VERSUS NURSES' KNOWLEDGE AND SKILLS

As educators, we have to analyze the present situation where nurses are so busy and proud with the rapid advances in technology that they tend to neglect the essence of nursing, which is ethics. It has been observed that nursing students enter school with a spirit of altruism, kindness, humanity, sensitivity, and a feeling for the dignity of human beings. They often have a definite, if naive, sense of right and wrong, and seem to be genuinely concerned with the moral and ethical consequences of their actions. However, somewhere along the line after graduation, these concerns and values are repressed enough that they are no longer present at a conscious level in professional functioning. Many nurses have been described as uncaring, insensitive, and hardened to the needs of their patients. Fromer (1981) describes these nurses as "not seeming to care about the social and ethical ramifications of professional practice" (p. xi). A number of factors seem responsible for this deteriorating sensitivity.

- Nurses are exposed so continually to such massive doses of human suffering that they seem to develop a sort of escape from suffering, which may result from having been taught how to deal with it realistically and effectively. It becomes easier to ignore a person's pain than to acknowledge it and face the fact that the nurse may have only limited resources to alleviate the pain.
- Health care delivery is moving toward becoming a scientific technology and gradually away from being a human art. It concentrates on disease rather on people, and on machines rather than on souls. Health professionals cannot help but be caught up in this scientific and technological fervor, which does not provide a favorable climate for ethical introspection.
- The curricula of nursing programs place emphasis on the physical senses

as well as the humanities. However, in actual clinical training experiences, there is a stress on the quantitative delivery of health care, which sets the stage for eventual diminution in importance of a sense of ethics. Therefore, ethics in nursing is limited to theoretical subjects that find little place in practical application, and do not serve to guide behavior and decisionmaking.

- The nature of the work that the nurses do in hospitals, in community health agencies, and in private practice leaves them little time to think about human values. A hospital nurse is too involved in attending to the physical needs of many patients and is frequently too exhausted to think of the ethical considerations of what she is doing. A community health nurse who spends all day racing from one client's home to another's together with hours at a crowded clinic is not going to have much time or energy for quiet reflection.

TEACHING STRATEGIES FOR THE SERVICE OF ETHICS

Educators should develop teaching strategies that will help student nurses to actually practice, rather than study, ethics, as they will learn through actually experiencing the autonomy, justice, veracity, fidelity, beneficence to do good, nonmaleficence to do harm, and paternalism. Education will be assimilated through proper tools of communication in teaching. Communication needs to be informative, open, and direct. The way a message is communicated is often as important as the word. According to Ney (1991), "An assertive communication is needed, without confrontation or accusing elements, is most effective when ethical problems are concerned" (p. 5).

It could follow the hierarchy given by Gilbert (1987):

1) *Receptivity* or *attention*: sensitivity to the existence of a certain phenomenon and includes a willingness to receive. Example: Noticing the anxiety of a patient awaiting the result of a laboratory test for a disease that can have serious consequences.

2) The second level is that of *response*. This implies sufficient interest in the phenomenon noticed to do something about it. Example: In the case described in the previous example, the response would be to say a few reassuring words to the patient so that he does not feel alone.

3) The third level is that of *internalization*. This implies that the perception of a phenomenon has found a place in one scale of values and has affected the person long enough for her to adapt herself to the value system of the other person. Example: On the death of a child, the attitude of the nurse

to members of his family will show them that she cares about their grief and is ready to help them to get over it. This means that the nurse has internalized the attitude that enables her to offer effective help.

Finally, the domain of ethics should be included in all nursing teaching. Student nurses should live the experience of practicing ethics until they reach the internalization of the values of nursing. In this way teaching will be more pervasive and will lead to positive changes in behavior.

REFERENCES

Bandman, E. & Bandman, B. (1985). *Nursing ethics in the life span*. Norwalk, CT: Appleton-Century-Crofts.

Churchill, L. (1977). Ethical issues of a profession in transition. *American Journal of Nursing, 77*, 873.

Fordham, M. (1992). In J. Brooking, S. Ritters, & B. Thomas, (Eds.), *A textbook of psychiatric and mental health nursing*, Ethics chapter (p. 69). Edinburgh: Churchill Livingstone.

Fromer, M. (1981). *Ethical issues in health care*. St. Louis: Mosby.

Gilbert, J. (1987). *Educational handbook for health personnel*. (6th ed.). Geneva: World Health Organization.

Harris, E. (1968). Respect for persons, in R. T. de George (Ed.), *Ethics and society: Original essays on contemporary moral problems* (pp. 111–132). New York: Macmillan.

Ney, C. (1991): *Nursing Ethics Resolution of Role Conflicts, Point of View*. Vol. 28 No. 1.

Patridge, K. (1978). Nursing values in a changing society. *Nursing Outlook, 6*, 356.

CHAPTER 14

Management Education for Nurses in the United States

Sheila A. Ryan, RN, PhD, FAAN, and
Colleen Conway-Welch, RN, PhD, CNM, FAAN

Bridging the knowledge, skills, and values of the corporate and professional domains demands an ever increasing knowledge of the business of health care. This chapter includes a discussion of the evolution of educational pathways for nursing executive development in the United States in the following areas:

1) Need for nurses with business skills;
2) History of education in nursing administration;
3) Commonwealth Fund dual degree initiative; and
4) Career and personal issues of nurses with Master's in Business Administration (MBA) degrees.

EMPLOYER NEED

Reform of the American health care system is underway and accelerating. The imposition of market forces, legislative imperatives, and management sophistication will lead the restructuring efforts in order to produce universal access to less costly health care for all Americans. The health care industry has been following the lead of the other giant, dominant United States corporations and global companies where past successes look increasingly like gross excesses.

Common areas for improvement include inefficient product or work quality, slow response to change with the marketplace, lack of innovation in work design and systems delivery, noncompetitive cost structure, inadequate employee involvement, unresponsive customer service, and inefficient and hierarchical, bureaucratic resource allocation. Each and all of these areas are basically management-induced and management-directed (Pearson, 1992).

All across corporate landscaping, corrective programs are being introduced, focused on operational improvements in quality, customers and costs, reallocating resources to their core business, and strategic planning for innovative work redesign.

121

In essence, managers have to change . . . have to change the organization; managers have to reinvent the values and goals toward which people strive, the ways people approach their work, the pace of the work in the organization, and how people work together. Managers have to organize people focused on change; managers have to institutionalize a totally new work environment. What will be required for these changes? Solutions include: Deciding unique and competitive corporate identities; setting higher performance standards; creating reward systems that reward performance and continuous improvement; and involving workers in the substance and work design aspects of the business, not just the administrative components.

Nurse executives continue to experience an increase in responsibilities and influence in both the broad institutional and extrainstitutional settings. They have accountability in the United States for 40% of the full time equivalents (FTE's) workers employed by hospitals and approximately 35% of most hospital operating budgets. The average nursing budget was reported to be $37.5 million (U.S.) in 1986 but ranges from $5 million to $333 million (U.S.). This average number of nursing FTEs is 658, but FTE's over 1000 are not uncommon. Top executive salaries for chief nursing officers in large institutions reach $150,000 (U.S.) (Mark, Turner, & Englehardt, 1990, p. 186).

Hospitals are restructuring work teams to cope with the sicker patient population. Also, senior nurse executives are being assigned larger areas of responsibility beyond nursing. Integrated systems for health delivery across settings requires knowledge and accountability for ambulatory practice, neighborhood clinics, home health, rehabilitative same-day surgery sites, and long-term care programs.

Along with increased levels of responsibility come some concerns about job security. Hospitals and organizations are dealing with restructuring, increasing efficiency, and significant economic downsizing. These factors may jeopardize some senior nurse executives' positions unless they are prepared to help their institutions with mergers, closings, and administrative restructuring.

Historically, organizations have relied on preparation for managers with strategies such as continuing education, trial and error, on the job training, mentoring/coaching, and internal training programs. This is no longer adequate to prepare nurse managers on the unit and interinstitutional level to cope with *changes* in:

- scope of practice;
- role responsibilities;
- organizational relationships;
- mix of professional and nonlicensed personnel;
- decentralization of authority;

- chains of command;
- management and philosophy; and
- morale and productivity requirements.

In addition, nurse executives and managers need to: use and manipulate data to justify cost and quality with patient care outcomes; initiate and manage program developments; develop and work with nursing/patient information systems; and incorporate research issues of outcome analysis and practice variations into daily patient care planning.

Expansion in both scope of practice and complexity of roles have caused the nurse manager and executive to need advanced analytical skills including preparation in financial management, marketing, computer information systems, and human resources management, in addition to health policy and quality outcome analysis, nursing theory and legal scope of practice issues, and nursing research methodologies.

As the scope of responsibilities expand, nurse managers and nurse executives become spokespersons for the profession and for key health issues in their political communities. The most significant responsibility, however, is the creation and maintenance of an environment within which professional nursing can be practiced.

The primary difference between nurse executives and nurse managers as suggested by Mark, Turner, and Englebardt (1990) is not the skills and knowledge difference but rather the focus. They suggested nurse executives focused on interinstitution and extrainstitution issues, where nurse managers focused on unit and intrainstitutional issues. It is the authors' contention that nurse executives and nurse managers share the same need for expanded business knowledge and increased understanding of the organizing and financing of changing health care systems.

HISTORY OF EDUCATION IN NURSING ADMINISTRATION

The first educational program in nursing administration was at Teacher's College, New York City, in 1899. It was not until the late 1940s that 13 universities developed graduate programs in nursing with the help of Kellogg Foundation funding. These programs were developed with a role focus minor in one of three functions: teaching, clinical specialist, or nursing administration. By the late 1970s, 24 universities (or approximately one-third of the universities with graduate nursing programs) offered a major in nursing administration. There was, however, increasing disenchantment in the profession towards promoting graduate education for clinical advancement, so functional preparation in teaching and administration declined. There are presently over 250 graduate programs in nursing with 74 programs offering nursing administration majors as well as clinical majors.

An analysis of graduate nursing administration programs by Stepura and Tilbury (1988) revealed that nursing administration curricula emphasized theory and research, especially administrative and organizational theory. Typically, generic course content consisted of nurse theory, theory development, professional issues, leadership, health care systems, and role theories. Yet the functions of executives and middle managers, and first-line managers include budget preparation and analysis decisionmaking, human resource allocation, and dealing with legal and ethical issues, as well as organizing, guiding, directing, evaluating, hiring, and firing.

The business skills required of today's nurse executive include: cost accounting, trend and variance analysis, human resource management, strategic planning, systems analysis, and marketing for more effective recruitment and retention. All the while, nurse executives must understand health, illness, and patient care issues across several settings that will enhance the effectiveness of resource allocation decisions. Nurse managers play a key role in how nurses practice and how the professional will advance.

A survey of nurse executive effectiveness by Moore, Biordi, Holm, and McElmurry (1988) compared characteristics of CNO effectiveness between chief executive officers (CEO) and CNOs from community hospitals. They compared their findings with an earlier study by Freund (1985), comparing CNO and CEO expectations of nurse effectiveness from university-owned hospitals. Top-ranking characteristics from both groups agreed on these top features: (a) human management skills; (b) total organizational view (more important to the CEOs than to the CNOs); (c) general management, general health, and nursing knowledge; (d) CEO's support (which the CNOs ranked highest); and lastly, (e) flexibility, negotiation, and compromise. In addition, Scalzi and Anderson (1989) reported that the overwhelming first choice of both of these groups for best preparation for nurse executives was the Masters Degree in Nursing plus MBA: 75% of CNOs and 65% of CEOs favored this over other choices, including MSN in administration, minors, majors, or a PhD.

THE COMMONWEALTH FUND INITIATIVE

The Commonwealth Fund, a U.S. philanthropic foundation based in New York City, sought to provide future nursing leaders with the same caliber of management, financial, and analytic training usually reserved for the business world, as health care is one of the nation's largest industries with expenses approaching $930 billion a year (U.S. dollars).

The Commonwealth Fund Board of Directors decided to support and promote the Master's in Business Administration (MBA) for nurses who already held a Master's in Nursing (MSN) in order to prepare these leaders. The Commonwealth Fund designed the Executive Nurse Fellowship and the recent initiatives to promote the MSN/MBA dual degree project. The Fund was established in 1918 by Anna M. Harkness to improve the common good of all, with emphasis on culturally diverse populations. The Fund has invested almost $6.5 million over the last 8 years for the development of nurse executives. The Fund believes that if the healthcare systems are to change, the nurse executive's role in these changes will be significant.

Approximately 150 awards (or fellowships) have been offered since 1986 to individual nurses pursuing their MBA, or combinations of degrees including the advanced management content. During 1987–89, the focus shifted to MBAs or joint programs for those with baccalaureate degrees in nursing. Initially, $25,000 was awarded to 15 applicants annually. That award level changed to $15,000 for 25 awardees annually. This project is now approaching its end as The Commonwealth Fund concluded the program had met its objectives.

DUAL DEGREE INITIATIVE

In the spring of 1989, The Commonwealth Fund's Advisory Committee of the Nurse Executive Fellowship Program discussed other ways to effect major change in the way nurse executives are educated and employed. The Commonwealth Fund awarded ten universities $100,000 each for a planning year to develop a joint MSN/MBA degree program. (Thirty-one universities were invited to submit proposals; 22 filed letters of intent, 22 applications were received, and 10 were funded for the academic year 1989–90.)

The Commonwealth Fund's Advisory Committee believes that the MSN/MBA degree can provide a career path for nurses into senior management. With the availability of the MSN/MBA degree and with prospects for a career in management, the nursing profession can also be far more attractive to groups of students who may not currently be considering nursing a career, but are looking at options such as law, medicine, or business. The joint degree can also entice college graduates without undergraduate nursing education to pursue graduate education in nursing and management. A number of the programs that are funded under this MSN/MBA arrangement also have some unique pathways for non-nurses to acquire their undergraduate nursing content and move directly into their Master's.

Common issues faced by these 10 programs during the planning years included curriculum issues, marketing and recruitment issues, admission requirement issues, and, obviously, financing issues.

Regarding the curriculum, the Commonwealth Fund's goal was to maintain quality while reducing the time to complete the MSN and MBA and to enhance integration between the schools of business and the schools of nursing. Most of the MSN programs were three to four semesters in length averaging 40 credits. Most of the MBA programs were at least four semesters with a range of 60 to 70 credits, on average. With this integration the majority of the MSN/MBA programs are five to six semesters, averaging a total of 76 credits. Hence, there is an economy of time with shared courses and reducing courses with common material.

Other issues of concern that still remain are marketing the program, the school, and recruitment into the dual track option. Some schools used the traditional ways of advertising in nursing journals and mail-out brochures; some schools conducted surveys to identify successful marketing efforts; others looked at financial assistance. Even though there is great interest in part-time study, the program's focus was to provide the financial resources to allow students to matriculate full time.

Procedures for admitting the applicant to the joint program vary across the different schools. Some have joint review committees; some have separate review committees; some have joint application processes. Some schools have a single admission to the joint program; others admit a single applicant to two separate programs. Many schools have separate issues that can only be settled according to each institutional preference.

Educational financing is a major issue in the United States. Nurses cannot afford to give up their income for three years, continue to raise families, and pay full-time tuition. Schools of nursing are continuing to look for corporate sponsorship and for hospital fellowships. It is a problem for many students to attend full-time, even with a scholarship. Some hospitals are not willing to allow an employee to take a leave of absence to complete a program full-time (and still hold their position). Pay-back arrangements are viable alternatives.

In summary, dual degree option provides students with strong management preparation including knowledge of:

- accounting;
- organizational behavior;
- human resource management;
- marketing;
- finance;
- information systems;
- advanced general knowledge in nursing; and
- application of research and theory to the administrative practice domain.

Problems of dual degree programs:

- Involvement of two separate schools, each having its own faculty, curriculum, administration, admissions criteria, marketing and recruitment efforts, and financing efforts;

- Coordination of admissions and course scheduling; and
- Maintenance and strengthening of the emphasis on nursing content throughout the dual degree program.

The nursing component is designed to provide a broad knowledge base of the practice and discipline components of professional nursing and their relationship to theory and research. The business component must help the student apply these to the administrative and financial domain.

CAREER AND PERSONAL ISSUES OF NURSE MBAs

In 1989, Lou Harris Survey, Inc. was contracted by Commonwealth to conduct a survey of nurse MBAs. Telephone interviews were conducted with over 300 nurse MBAs, which was believed to be a substantial portion of the population. A convenience sample approaching the full population was gathered by inviting schools to share their graduation lists. Heretofore, there had not been a directory or inventory of nurse MBAs. Although the survey queried participants about experiences prior to, during and after the MBA, reasons for the MBA, applying to and perceived benefits, only a few questions, regarding the MSN/MBA are reported here.

Although 66% were satisfied with nursing as a career before starting an MBA, the most frequently mentioned reason for choosing to enter was the desire to increase career options. Over half wanted to stay within nursing. Seventy percent were interested in choices other than nursing, if the opportunities sounded right. Many nurse MBAs stated as their main reason a desire to increase skills applicable to nursing. Over half said it was very important to have the necessary skills to advance in the profession; and several of them said they needed it for their current position to do a better job. Additionally, over half said the MBA was very important in order to increase their salary. In 1989, the median yearly income prior to getting their MBA was $28,600.

Over half of the nurses surveyed were full-time MBA students. Yet, over 94% worked while going to school and raising a family. The mean of their working hours was 40 hours per week. For women in the 1990s, these are the issues: working, expanding, raising children, and developing careers.

How was their education financed? Over half (54%) received educational financing from their employer. Of these, 58% of their tuition was paid by their employer. So, a significant reason why people worked full-time while pursuing their MBA was for the financial assistance.

Over three-fourths (75%) said the MBA was very important in getting their current job. Almost 90% said it was important in doing their job well. In addition, almost 80% reported that their clinical skills contributed to their credibility in their position. (Over 70% said their clinical skills contributed to their effectiveness regardless of their management position.) Even with the MBA degree, there is a strong conviction that both advanced clinical preparation and management skills are essential. Forty-six percent are still in their first post-MBA job with the same employer. But 64% left their post-MBA job for another.

The MBA has proved financially rewarding for many. The median starting salary of their first post-MBA job yielded a $6,000 increase on average. The current median salary, compared with salaries prior to the MBA, represents a $15.7 thousand dollar raise or a 40% increase pre- to post-MBA position.

Almost all (88%) would advise other nurses to pursue an MBA, and over 60% would be willing to help and advise. Almost all of them would be interested in networking with each other for career and professional reasons.

CLOSING

A combined MSN/MBA seems to offer career opportunities, career mobility, and a way to retain nurses in nursing. There are some benefits, particularly in both salary and satisfaction to young professionals on the move. More specifically, it will be important to show that with the advances in health care, the opportunities and expanding roles and responsibilities, nurse executives will play a key part in shaping the future of health delivery.

Nurses with a combined MSN/MBA can bring many benefits to the profession. They are compensated well and are knowledgeable in entrepreneurial and intrapreneurial activities. They are skilled in analyzing outcomes of practice variations and can identify and bring new nursing "products" to the marketplace. Finally, their expertise in information systems development makes them valuable members of interdisciplinary teams.

These "new" nurses reflect a shift in educational content from discipline-specific content to broader content including critical thinking, collaboration, shared decision making and analyses, and interventions at systems/aggregate levels.

To summarize, in order to survive in tomorrow's world and claim a leadership position, our educational systems must produce graduates who are skilled in reading and understanding business journals as well as nursing journals.

REFERENCES

Freund, C. M. (1985). Director of nursing effectiveness. *Journal of Nursing Administration, 15*, 25–30.

Mark, B. A., Turner, J. T., & Englebardt, S. (1990). Knowledge and skills for nurse administrators. *Nursing and Health Care, 11*, 184–189.

Moore, K., Biordi, K., Holm, K., & McElmurry, B. (1988). Nurse executive effectiveness. *Journal of Nursing Administration, 18*, 23–27.

Pearson, A. (1992). Corporate redemption and the seven deadly sins. *Harvard Business Review, 70*, 65–75.

Scalzi, C. C., & Anderson, R. A. (1989). Dual degree: Future preparation for nurse executives? *Journal of Nursing Administration, 19*, 25–9.

Stepura, B. A., & Tilbury, M. S. (1988). An analysis of academic programs preparing nurse administrators. *Journal of Nursing Administration, 18*, 8.

CHAPTER 15

Computers in Nursing Education

Marianne Tallberg, RN, PhD

T his chapter will discuss computer literacy, computer based or assisted learning, and integration of the use of computers in the nursing curriculum. Even though the author has attempted a global approach to the topic, the perspective presented is much influenced by the state of the art in Finland and Europe.

> Nursing Informatics is the use of nursing science, computer science and information science in nursing processes for patient/client care which provides data, information and knowledge to the individual and the organization in such a way as to enhance health in society whilst protecting the individual and achieving health for all. (International Medical Informatics Association, 1992 minutes from Geneva meeting, p. 4)

Still, this definition does not include the strict educational use of computers, so it has to be amended.

> True computer literacy is not just knowing how to make use of computers and computational ideas. It is knowing when it is appropriate to do so. (Papert, 1980, p. 155)

In many parts of the world "computers in nursing" is taught as a separate course, if it is taught at all, in the nursing schools. That makes nurses look at computers as something insignificant and sometimes also dangerous for nursing. When integrating the use of computers in all parts of nursing education, they should be shown as a useful tool for nurses.

Dreyfus and Dreyfus (1986) have created the model of the five steps, from novice to expert, that Benner (1984, pp. 13–38) has used so cleverly in showing how nurses learn their skills. When adapting those steps to nurses' "computer literacy", it is regrettable that many nurses stop at the second stage, that of advanced beginner, i.e., their performance improves only to a marginally acceptable level. For reached "competence" Dreyfus and Dreyfus request that one should no longer merely follow designed rules which means that one should at least be able to take shortcuts in the program or use other efficiency-improving techniques. This is not very common. Some nurses reach "proficiency," but there are few that can be called "experts." This deficiency is affecting the whole health care area in Europe. There has not been sufficient research on the educational process of teaching and learning in the use of computers. The special needs of the various health care professionals must direct their preparation.

The Council of Europe Committee of Ministers agreed in 1990 on a recommendation on training strategies for health information systems. The main purpose of the recommendation is that the member states:

- ensure that, as soon as possible, those staff involved in health care receive appropriate multidisciplinary training, both theoretical and practical, for health information systems within an overall public health context
- develop training strategies for health information systems, which take account of their overall development and of the organization and circumstances of local health
- establish international co-operation through a network of reference centers, in order to facilitate the exchange of knowledge and resources in a new and rapid changing field (Council of Europe Committee of Ministers, 1990, p. 1).

The European Community program "Advances in Medical Informatics" has answered this challenge and started a Concerted action (CA) on education and training in health care informatics (Advances in Medical Informatics Program [AIM], 1992). The aim of the CA is to create computer literacy model curricula for different health care professionals. Several professionals throughout Europe are involved in this project. The final proposals will be presented during 1994.

COMPUTER-BASED EDUCATION (CBE)

What is CBE about? It is not so easily defined because of a growing market of new categories of educational computer programs. For the umbrella term of hypermedia/multimedia we can use the following definition:

> User led programs through linkage of sound, pictures, text, graphics, and animation via interconnecting windows on a particular subject area. (Heimburger & Kuhanen, 1993, p. 327)

How frequent is the use of computer-based educational programs in nursing education? If one looks at it globally it is impossible to give an exact answer. But one can draw the conclusion that there is an increasing interest by looking at the amount of articles on this topic. In the 1970s it was nearly impossible to find an article on the subject in any journal—educational, technical, and certainly not in nursing journals. Moving into the 1980s the journal "Computers in Nursing" was launched, but educational use of computers was seldom referred to (Gnobe, 1984). An interest began to arouse first with the microcomputer boom in the middle and late 1980s. Today, scarcely a nursing educational or nursing computer journal issue appears without at least some comments on the subject.

Drilling and Writing

Among the first programs to enter the nursing educational world were Computer Managed Instruction (CMI) programs. In this type of programs the computer restricts the student to a certain point. Teacher-designed pretests and student evaluation programs are two examples of fields of application. This group of drill and practice programs has been popular in supporting students in mathematics, especially to providing training on drug dose calculation. Otherwise, this category of programs has been looked at as too monotonous and repetitive.

The computer is a very effective and efficient tool for word processing. Until now, particularly viewing nursing education from a Finnish viewpoint, writing essays and writing on the whole has had a too limited part in the nurse education. The computer with a good word processing program could help to change teaching methods. Writing exercises will also constitute an element in the computer literacy preparation by getting nurses accustomed to computers.

Computer-Assisted Learning and Expert Systems

Computer-Assisted learning (CAL) programs are those in which the program is constructed for facilitating the students' learning. These programs should leave space for the student to use the program for his/her own learning purposes.

From a variety of definitions the following has been chosen because it looks at "computer-assisted learning" from an outcome standpoint.

> A relatively permanent change in skills, knowledge or attitudes stimulated by one or more interactions between the individual and the computer. (James & Turner, 1992, p. 10)

Intelligent tutoring systems provide training in clinical judgement when simulations provide an opportunity to expose the student to more unusual events. By using knowledge-based expert systems, students could exercise their critical thinking, and learn how to solve problems and make decisions in a safe environment.

Interactive Video and Virtual Reality

While simulation is an ideal method for teaching clinical nursing, it is a resource-consuming method. Here computer simulations have a future. Interactive video (IV) is a videodisc player linked to a personal computer with a program developed for interactive learning use. Using the IV, the students can be presented with realistic simulations of various situations. The program provides the student with the possibility to administer care to the factive patient without causing harm. The program gives feedback about the students' achievement.

Virtual reality is the latest hypermedia construction and is really a step further from IV. It has been defined as

> a highly interactive, computer-based, multimedia environment in which the user becomes a participant with the computer in a "virtually real" world (Pantelidis, 1993, p. 23).

Philips asks in an article in *Nursing Science Quarterly* if virtual reality will be a new vista for nurse researchers? (Phillips, 1993). It will certainly be a much more "alive" simulation environment when students really can "go in" and administer care to virtual patients. Perhaps this can be the future way to prepare professionals for caregiving in a laboratory setting.

Bulletin Boards and Databases

The increased use of electronic mail has opened many new possibilities. The communication is not limited to the internal network in nursing schools; contact to the outside world is open through international networks. Nursing associations and educational authorities are establishing nursing bulletin boards for nursing students, teachers, and practicing nurses to exchange opinions of common interest.

Through the international networks it is possible to use the "Gopher" system for searching literature in libraries throughout the world. Databases for searching nursing literature have also come nearer to students with the expanding use of CD-ROM, saving many countries the high costs of online retrieval.

EVALUATING AND SELECTING OF EDUCATIONAL PROGRAMS

Evaluation of a computer-assisted learning package's significance for nursing education requires a nurse teacher well acquainted not only with the goals for the course where the package will be used, but also with the whole nursing curriculum and the school's philosophy. At the same time, the teacher requires some overall guidelines to help her with this task. Burke (1993) asserts that in the UK there is nationally no unified or structured plan for the use, development or evaluation of CAL. She is really stressing a very significant point, "the national view," because one has to be aware of cultural differences even though the language may be the same. In Europe a common decree about nursing education is being developed but it will not totally remove the cultural differences within health care. Burke also identified the lack of evaluation instruments, as an issue and Sparks (1990) of the National Library of Medicine Learning Center has already commented on this deficiency.

In a review of evaluation instruments published in 1993, the reviewers (Sparks & Kuenz, 1993) criticize the evaluators for misuse of their responding audience by asking irrelevant questions. They comment also on the evaluation's lack of validity. The most important criterion for evaluation should be the philosophical and curricular fit, and the matching of technological requirements with the institution's capabilities.

Another matter to be aware of is the computer interface. With the growing Human-Computer Interaction research we can demand a computer interface that is suitable to our needs (Koivunen, 1993). In deciding what teaching material to use, the humanistic view on the teacher as facilitator must predominate. In humanistic didactic the computer must always be steered by people, used as a tool and a servant.

COMPUTER PROGRAMS' SIGNIFICANCE FOR NURSE EDUCATION

How should we acquire the best effect when integrating the use of CAL and other hypermedia tools in our curricula? Many comments on computer-supported programs support a new curriculum revolution which takes the multimedia methods into consideration from the beginning (Seels, 1993). Changing to a process-driven curriculum instead of the traditional content-driven curriculum leads to a peer relationship between student and faculty and changes the students' attitudes and liability for the outcome (Marcinek, 1993). This new perspective on teaching requires multimedia as method and tool. This is true even one respects the view quoted from *Technology 2001* that expressed the means of enhancing education are not going to be technological (Leebaert & Dickinson, 1991).

DISCUSSION

How can one explain the fact that the use of hypermedia still has to struggle for full acceptance? Are the teachers anxious about their replacement? If so, they have misunderstood the use of computers in education.

It has been quite common to use CAL as a learning strategy to help students with difficulties in keeping pace with their fellow students. Mostly those students are from an ethnic minority group with language difficulties, but other students with a deficient educational background have also taken advantage of CAL (Goodman, Blake, & Lott, 1990; Lerner, Cohen, & Brown, 1992). Frequently used under these conditions CAI has perhaps led to a distorted report of some programs. Maybe this use has misled some teachers to think that CAI is not something for their brave ordinary students.

In nursing education one can differentiate between two teaching aims, i.e., skills teaching and knowledge teaching, but these also have to be integrated. When using information technology in education, one has to go beyond a didactic view, solving learning problems by using learning theories. This has many times been forgotten; the CAL has not been integrated in the curriculum with careful afterthought.

There are many positive factors associated with hypermedia. For example, students can set their own pace; the program can be repeated as often as required; and a standard can be set in a topic area. Working independently gives the student the potential to achieve broader objectives and complete multifaceted assignments. The students can plan their studies and styles depending on experience and plans for the future. On the other hand, an individual studying independently has to be self-confident and have good inner motivation, and be systematic, open to experiments, curious, flexible, and persistent under stress. Such a student has to be self-governing and dauntless for being able to set his/her own aims and choose the methods differing from conventional views.

the new technology is a challenge for the faculty. Curriculum building depends on their broad view and didactic knowledge. In the process-driven curriculum, with vast independence for the students, it requires of the faculty an innovative approach to student monitoring.

REFERENCES

Advances in Medical Informatics Program. (1992). *Concerted Action on teaching and training: Preparatory workshop*. Brussels: Author.

Burke, L. (1993). Effective evaluation of CAL software packages. *Information Technology in Nursing, 5*, 5–7.

Council of Europe Committee of Ministers. (1990). *Recommendation No. R (90) 21*. Strasbourg, France: Author.

Dreyfus, H. L., & Dreyfus, S. E. (1986). *Mind over machine: The power of human intuition and expertise in the era of the computer*. New York: The Free Press.

Goodman, J., Blake, J., & Lott, M. (1990). CAI: A strategy for retaining minority and academically disadvantaged students. *Nurse Educator, 15*, 37–41.

Grobe, S. J. (1984). *Computer primer and resource guide for nurses*. Philadelphia: Lippincott.

Heimburger, A., & Kuhanen, T. (1993). Hypermedia. In E. Hyvönen, I. Karanta, & M. Syrjänen (Eds.), *Tekoälyn ensyklopedia* (pp. 327–333). Helsinki: Gaudeamus.

International Medical Informatics Association. (1992). *Working Group 8 meeting report*. Geneva: Author.

James, M. E., & Turner, P. (1992). Computer assisted learning. *Information Technology in Nursing, 4*, 10–11.

Koivunen, M–R. (1993). Ihminen ja tietokoneen vuorovaikutus [ ]. In E. Hyvönen, I. Karanta, & M. Syrjänen (Eds.), *Tekoälyn ensyklopedia* (pp. 319–326). Helsinki: Gaudeamus.

Leebaert, D., & Dickinson, T. (1991). A world to understand: Technology and the awakening of human possibility. In D. Leebaert (Ed.), *Technology 2001: The future of computing and communications* (pp. 293–321). Cambridge: The MIT Press.

Lerner, H., Cohen, B., & Brown, M. (1992). Computer usage among high-risk baccalaureate nursing students. In J. M. Arnold & G. A. Pearson (Eds.), *Computer applications in nursing education and practice* (pp. 207–215). New York: National League for Nursing.

Marcinek, M. A. (1993). The curriculum revolution: Transforming barriers to education for registered nurses. *Nurse Educator, 18*, 13–16.

Pantelidis, V. S. (1993). Virtual reality in the classroom. *Educational Technology, 33*, 23–27.

Papert, S. (1980). *Mindstorms: Children, computers and powerful ideas*. Brighton: The Harvester Press.

Phillips, J. R. (1993). A new vista for nurse researchers? *Nursing Science Quarterly, 6*, 5–7.

Seels, B. (1993). The view looking back: Curriculum theory and instructional technology programs. *Educational Technology, 33*, 2127.

Sparks, S. (1990). Computer-based education in nursing. Lister Hill Monograph LHNCBC 90–1). Washington, DC: U.S. Department of Health and Human Services.

CHAPTER 16

Re-Entry of Students

Diane McGivern, RN, PhD, FAAN

I n my position as Head of the Division of Nursing at New York University in the United States I hear many stories from nurses about their career plans, unexpected career changes, and need for career guidance. Frequently the conversations revolve around some precipitating event which makes them seriously consider returning to school to complete their degree requirements. Sometimes these stories are sad—such as when re-entry to nursing education is prompted by the loss of a job or loss of a spouse. Sometimes the notion of returning to school is an exciting adventure which has been delayed by raising children or living in a remote area of the country.

In most fields, re-entering students are becoming the standard and not the exception. Career change and mobility have become the norm as people live longer, economic conditions fluctuate, and the demand for products and services change rapidly. The legal retirement age and other perceived limits on work life are rapidly disappearing.

Re-entering or returning students are certainly not a new phenomenon in nursing education. Hospital-based diploma and associate degree programs continue to produce graduates while at the same time personal, social, and professional forces are prompting nurses to return to colleges and universities to earn degrees in nursing and other disciplines (Innes & Oulton, 1990). Nursing programs in a number of countries have had several decades to develop and test education models for these nontraditional students.

At the same time, the groups that re-entering nursing students are joining are not homogenous either. Increasingly, baccalaureate programs attract students with academic and experiential preparation in other fields, older full-time workers with no higher education, and current college students with a change of heart about their original choices. The health care field, and nursing in particular, can benefit from the diversity of this applicant pool, because the postbasic nurses and others bring judgment born of varied life experiences and a commitment to gaining more education.

There is universal agreement that the international nursing community, and those it serves, need nurses with postbasic education who are prepared to meet worldwide primary health care needs, create social change, and contribute to the economy through the health and education sectors.

Education research on the needs of re-entering students has shifted over time from an examination of student and educational program characteristics to research on conceptual and unifying views of health professions education, primary health care, and a systems change which is cost-effective, efficient, and productive of desired health outcomes.

The next phase of educational research should focus on three areas: (a) collaboration among educators, administrators, and practitioners, to produce a leadership culture, (b) continued technological development which reflects input of nursing and general educators, and (c) the national development of well-articulated postbasic and graduate nursing education programs which reflect local health and cultural expectations.

SIGNIFICANCE

Why is the re-entering student population so important to the international community of nurses? There are three reasons re-entry students require special attention: (a) in many countries they will be the new proponents of primary care; (b) they are the potential candidates for future faculty positions; and lastly, (c) they are a part of the country's economic growth.

We subscribe to the belief that baccalaureate and higher degree education provides the knowledge and skills basic to strong professional socialization (Woodman, Knecht, Periard, & Bell, 1991), enhanced leadership capability, and a broader understanding of individual as well as community health care needs.

And while the statistics on nurse preparation, licensure, registration, and postregistration education are not readily available from many countries, empirical evidence suggested that many countries are planning and implementing basic, re-entry, and baccalaureate education programs which address national primary health care needs, faculty development for programs which support clinical and research activity, and ways in which the health care sector will contribute to the overall economy. Re-entry nurses are vital to these three initiatives.

Primary Care

In order to meet the international goal of Health for All by the year 2000 (Declaration at Alma Ata) practitioners in every country need to be recruited to, and prepared in, programs which stress scientifically based clinical preparation; competence in primary, secondary, and tertiary care; and professional practice which reflects equity and respect among health care professionals and government officials. The 1978 International Conference on Primary Health Care and 1981 World Health Assembly adopted the goal of health for all and noted that nursing was key to meeting this vital goal of health for all.

Primary care is characterized by five principles: universal coverage; continuum of promotive, preventive, curative, rehabilitative, and long-term services; services that are accessible, affordable, and culturally acceptable; those that are community-focused; and those related to other economic sectors. Hirschfield (Hirschfield & Holleran, 1992) points out that in order to meet the challenge of primary care for all, nursing must bring together its education, practice, and management sectors to produce sound education and improved practice.

The goals of nursing education must be consistent with the goals to provide health care to every citizen. Advanced education is desirable because it provides the strong professional socialization needed by nurses who will provide the leadership, expand the theoretical and experiential base necessary for practice, and prepare other nurses to manage the rapid technological advances not only with manual dexterity but also with the appreciation of the ethical, economic, and moral implications.

Many international writers agree with Osei-Boateng (1992, p. 176) who, writing about her own home, Africa, asserts: "Nursing education (in Africa) should prepare the polyvalent nurse who can function in all settings to meet the total health care needs of individuals, families, and communities within the framework of the primary health care program." (p. 196).

Inherent in our aspirations for primary health care for all are educational goals which rest on the considerable body of literature about change. Writers agree that advanced education is needed to promote change (Ehrente, German, & Zir, 1992). Many describe the role of education as empowering nurses to change the social environment, empower the people they serve, and effect improvements in local and national health policy (Abugharbien & Suliman, 1992; Clay, 1992).

Faculty Preparation

Through education re-entry students have opportunities to gain broader theoretical understanding of primary care, analyze the determinants of national health policy, and anticipate the nurse's role in multiprofessional efforts on behalf of people seeking care. Re-entry education also should strengthen their clinical practice, integrate the primary care component, and prepare them for leadership.

The second significance of re-entry students relates to faculty preparation. Re-entering students create the need both for additional faculty with advanced preparation and present themselves as potential candidates for the roles of advanced clinicians and academicians. Their value is enhanced by the hope that they will contribute to the cadre of educational program faculty. Therefore, they should be socialized to value and seek advanced education, and be prepared to design curricula relevant to community health, social needs, and the national development priorities. Two important components are resources and role-modeling. Library resources for faculty, re-entry and other students should be a combination of materials reflecting local practices and books and journals from abroad (Osei-Boateng, 1992). Faculty role-modeling is also essential to attract the most able re-entry students and to encourage their preparation for academic leadership.

Contribution to the Economy

Finally, re-entry students are important for their contributions to the economy. Nurses' re-entry into the education arena enhances education's and health care's contribution to the economy. Higher education results in better compensated positions, and stimulates the development of future products and services. Higher education for re-entry nurses which promotes cost-effective primary health care services also has clear economic benefits. To the extent that successful primary care initiatives are cost-effective, additional money may be available for education and health care. Higher education drives economic growth through university-based research which generates future developments and attracts additional public and private enterprise. Higher education also plays a significant role in interrupting the cycle of poverty, reducing welfare expenditures and contributing to state revenues. Higher education is important as a way to set and monitor standards for licensed professionals, thereby maintaining quality in health services delivery, which has an economic return as well.

EVOLUTION OF RE-ENTRY EDUCATION

In keeping with the importance of re-entry education, there has been and continues to be much published research on students and instructional issues. The educational research and curricular developments related to re-entry education in the late 1970s and the 1980s was focused somewhat narrowly on the special characteristics of adult students and the implications for the education program (Lengacher & Van Cott, 1992). The adult learner theories postulate that the older, nontraditional students, by virtue of their life experiences, maturity, significant work experience, and motivation require a different pedagogical approach from the allegedly more compliant secondary school graduates newly embarking on a college or training program. Knowles (1980), a key theorist, identified two conditions necessary for learning to take place. For the adult learner, the instructional situation has to reflect a climate of collaboration, mutual trust, and respect. At the same time, students must become active participants in planning their own educational objectives and learning experiences.

Student characteristics studied included learning styles, motivation, adult learner preferences, and developmental patterns (Mattson, 1990). The many factors which motivate students to return to nursing education programs were also investigated. Common motivating factors expressed by re-entry students and studied exhaustively were the desire for professional advancement, added knowledge, improvement in social welfare skills (Lethbridge, 1989), desire to attend graduate school, and access to higher level positions (Thurber, 1988). In a study of over 13,000 students in Africa, Asia, New Zealand, Canada, and the United States, six motivating factors included professional advancement, interest in learning, social stimulation, social contact, external expectations, and community service (Boshier & Collins, 1985). Other motivators identified through observation and experience included official requests from the ministers of health, hospital or agency administrators, or colleagues and mentors who directed or otherwise enticed nurses to gain postbasic education, usually with a very specific plan in mind.

The proposed conclusions of the studies on student characteristics served as bases for varied curriculum plans which were, in turn, also investigated (Baj, 1985; Ehrenfeld et al., 1992; Fraser & Titherington, 1991).

Much of the research assumed that the adult learner theories of Knowles and others would determine the structure of re-entry programs. But while re-entry programs differ around the world, they all intend to provide a "professionalizing" or professional "socializing" experience, one that is career-oriented, supports autonomy, and enhances intellectual growth and self-actualization.

A re-entry program may be a self-contained, second step or upper division program, or a traditional generic baccalaureate program with entry points for nontraditional students. In re-entry programs faculty have attempted to tailor course work to the different academic and experiential backgrounds, adopt appropriate teaching methodologies, create novel clinical learning experiences, and modify the negative attitudes of students which interfere with learning and resocialization.

However, subsequent research and considerable faculty and student experience have determined that re-entering students or adult learners were not necessarily conforming to Knowles' adult learner model (Burnard and Morrison, 1992; Ryan, 1985). A reviewer of the literature on nontraditional students concluded that although the use of adult learning concepts has been cited frequently in discussions of re-entry students, a lack of evidence remains to support the use of "andragogical" principles with adult nursing students. In fact, nursing research suggests that nontraditional students are not significantly different from traditional baccalaureate students in their preferences for instructional methods (Thompson, 1992). Unlike the predictions of the adult learner model, these students do not automatically know how to handle freedom and responsibility. Merritt (1983), for example, found that adult learners were less positively oriented toward the learning environment and methods, did not necessarily want to set their own goals, and preferred structure, definition, and organization.

Despite the educational and economic reasons to establish tailored re-entry programs responsive to students' needs, students have anticipated or actually encountered a number of obstacles to their education, including lack of program flexibility, inconvenient course scheduling, geographic inaccessibility of schools or instructional sites, and the duplications of nursing knowledge and experience from their first nursing training program (MacLean, 1985). Returning students identified difficulty in coordinating their work responsibilities and academic requirements, felt a lack of recognition of their previously mastered knowledge and skills, and experienced a lack of understanding of the required change in their professional socialization.

We must move on to a new phase of research on re-entry programs and focus on the next essential elements of re-entry education: distance learning, program linkages from technical preparation through master's study, and the development of leadership capability.

Re-Entry Research of the 1980s and 1990s

Just as the requirements of students and the profession are changing, the goals of higher education are also being reformulated to accommodate changing national demographics, national economic trends, and technological developments. The research focus of re-entry education began to expand somewhat in the late 1980s. In a review of North American nursing literature (Lengacher & Van Cott, 1992), 31 studies reflected the earlier interest in the personal characteristics and socialization of postbasic students, the curriculum and programmatic issues, as well as the newer interest in more innovative teaching/learning strategies. The latter research includes studies on parallel track programs (King, 1988), audio and teleconferencing (Dugas, 1985; Henry, 1993), and other long-distance teaching technologies (Cragg, 1991; Dirksen, 1993). Research on innovation and technology needs to be aggressively pursued since it holds the greatest promise for access to higher education, efficient use of resources, and enhanced programmatic quality.

We must move on to a new phase of research on re-entry programs and focus on the next essential elements of re-entry education: distance learning, program linkages from technical preparation through master's study, and the development of leadership capability.

Long-Distance Learning

Recognizing the importance of baccalaureate and higher degree programs for clinicians and faculty, many countries are devising ways to provide instructions to overcome the obstacles of 1) travel over significant distances (Cragg, 1991; Lorensen & Schej, 1992; Shomaker, 1993) and the harsh climate; and 2) multiple responsibilities of nurses (95% of whom are women); and in the current economy, the need to balance full-time work and an academic workload.

"Distance learning" is an innovative instructional tactic which provides information in ways other than the formal face-to-face situation. Distance education provides for collaboration among several geographically separate educational and clinical programs, each with unique strengths. This dramatically increases the variety and availability of theoretical and clinical content. Cost-effectiveness and time-efficiency are important outcomes of sending instruction from a central site to individuals or groups of students tens or thousands of miles away.

Distance learning capitalizes on a variety of technologies which may range from simple systems to more elaborate interactive capability. Two approaches are possible. The first attempts to simulate traditional, face-to-face classroom instruction. Groups of students meet together and may interact with a distant instructor and other groups of students at other sites. Audioteleconferencing is one such example.

A second approach is one in which individual learners study alone or on an individual timetable. Examples of this include correspondence courses which may supply written materials, audio- or videotapes, and/or telephone conferences with the instructor. One current multistate program provides opportunities for re-entry degree students to take videotaped courses using tapes delivered directly to the students' worksite. Tapes are supplemented by required papers, oral and written examinations, and counseling and advisement (Paulanka, 1993).

Related pedagogical issues under study include distance learning's impact on professional socialization (Cragg, 1991), on achievement, and the students' future contributions to professional nursing. Research is needed on the effectiveness of distance learning's integration of primary health care, interdisciplinary collaboration, and leadership strategies.

PROGRAM ARTICULATION

While the need for educational programs responsive to the needs of re-entering students is international in scope, programs should be unique in detail and requirements for each of the countries we represent. Many re-entering students cite the desire to gain master's degrees and enter advanced practice as the reason to return to nursing education programs. The real or perceived difficulty in moving from one level of preparation to another speaks to the need for national models of linkage between programs so that basic, postbasic baccalaureate, and master's program content build on each other with efficiency, cost-effectiveness, and relevance to national health care. These models may differ from country to country, depending on the availability of education for women, the history and future goals established for nursing education, and the national plan for health care and health professions education. The experience for Australia which just established collegiate education as the only model (Marquis, Lillibridge, & Madison, 1993) will be different from the United States (Fagin & Lynaugh, 1992), which will be different again from Jordan (AbuGharbich & Suliman, 1992) the Pacific Rim (Fritsch, 1992), Africa (Osei-Boateng, 1992), and elsewhere.

Educational mobility models have been hampered by lack of available resources, difficulty in establishing systems of evaluating previous learning (Lengacher & Van Cott, 1992), and some disagreement about whether the articulation concept should be a temporary measure until there is determination of a single model or standard of education (Fagin, 1990).

Credit for postbasic nursing courses is established through examination and in many cases is used to earn advanced placement in the upper division. These credits by examination and other forms of validation reflect a belief that there is shared content in basic and baccalaureate programs. Several states (including California, Minnesota, New Mexico, and Florida) have established statewide articulation plans to allow all postbasic graduates to directly transfer or obtain credit in baccalaureate programs.

A number of programs have been established in the United States to enable the postbasic graduate to complete both the baccalaureate and master's degree requirements in a coherent sequence. Two routes commonly followed are: establishment of credit for previously taken coursework or life experience, and a combination of post-basic and master's content which makes the baccalaureate degree requirement integral to master's programs (McHugh, 1991).

It is important to note that linkage or articulation programs which include master's preparation should demonstrate specialist education that is built on a foundation of generalist knowledge and skills.

LEADERSHIP

While there is universal agreement regarding the need for nurses to actively engage in policy debate, assess the need for and provide primary care, and assume responsibility for effecting change, educational programs are inconsistent in developing leadership content and differentiating among leadership expectations at the basic, postbasic baccalaureate, and master's degree levels. Responsibilities for policy formulation, leadership in interdisciplinary forums, and leadership in management positions demand particular skills and a broad base of knowledge in nurses with postbasic education.

In some settings, women are not expected to assume leadership roles, advocate for others in the community, or balance gender and occupational responsibilities. Leadership then requires not only skills but role modeling and empowerment in order for nurses who are women to take on these activities.

Leadership in the context of re-entry education begins with the selection of the *most able* students and progresses to a development of strong relationships among nursing policymakers, educators, and returning students. Nursing leadership must be enhanced by simultaneously sustaining the pioneers in nursing while developing the younger professionals who have the potential skill and share similar interests.

Collaboration and communication among nurses in various sectors and roles and at various career phases are achieved through initiatives such as joint appointments, collaborative research, mentorship programs, institutional and international partnership programs, and planned efforts to ensure that others succeed in organizational leadership.

Leadership training for all is enhanced by access to educational programs and experience which stress fiscal, regulatory, political, organizational, and management principles.

A MODEL

A number of programs for re-entering students have developed over the last three decades and provide national models. Many of these have successfully addressed students' concerns while adhering to established academic and professional standards. Successful programs are characterized by recognition of students' previous competencies, use of learning theories which recognize individual differences as central to curriculum development, and give special regard for students' present and future contributions.

One model of a re-entry program which has stimulated much discussion and controversy is the New York State Regents College Degrees in Nursing program. The program is based on the philosophy that the knowledge an individual possesses is more important than how the knowledge was acquired.

The re-entry baccalaureate degree program offered by Regents College is fully accredited; is a noninstructional, assessment-based, independent study program. It awards college level credits when individuals demonstrate college level proficiency by successfully completing a series of assessments in cognitive and skill components of nursing. The entire nursing component of the curriculum consists of examinations which, when satisfactorily completed, define end-point college level competencies and reflect the content of traditional baccalaureate programs.

While controversial, the Regents program has created access for large numbers of nurses and developed examinations now used by traditional institutionally based programs.

In summary, model programs for re-entry students are ones which:

- create access for the greatest numbers of students who meet admissions standards;
- assess and build on previous learning;
- provide generalist preparation;
- include theory and clinical practice which integrates primary care;
- prepare for leadership; and
- socialize students to seek advance preparation.

REFERENCES

AbuGharbieh, P., & Suliman, W. (1992). Changing the image of nursing in Jordan. *International Nursing Review, 39*, 149–152.

Baj, P. (1985). Can the generic curriculum function for the returning RN student? *Journal of Nursing Education, 24*, 69–71.

Boshier, R. W., & Collins, R. (1985). The Houle typology after twenty-two years: A large-scale empirical test. *Adult Education Quarterly, 35*, 113–130.

Burnard, P., & Morrison, P. (1992). Students' and lecturers' preferred teaching strategies. *International Journal Nursing Studies, 29*, 345–353.

Clay, T. (1992). Education and empowerment: Securing nursing's future. *International Nursing Review, 39*, 15–18.

Cragg, C. (1991). Professional resocialization of post-RN baccalaureate students by distance education. *Journal of Nursing Education, 30*, 256–260.

Dirksen, S. R. (1993). RN/BSN distance learning through microwave. *Nurse Educator, 18*, 13–17.

Dugas, B. W. (1985). Baccalaureate for entry to practice. *The Canadian Nurse, 81* 17–19.

Ehrenfeld, M., Bergman, R., & Ziv, L. 91992). Academia: A stimulus for change. *International Nursing Review, 39*, 23–26.

Fagin, C. (1990). Conference Overview. In C. Fagin (Ed.), *Nursing Leadership: Global Strategies* (pp. xiv–xxiv). New York: (National League for Nursing Publication No. 41-2349).

Fagin, C., & Lynaugh, J. (1992). Reaping the rewards of radical change: A new agenda for nursing education. *Nursing Outlook, 40*, 213–220.

Fraser, M., & Titherington, R. (1991). Where are they now? The career paths of graduates from post-registration degrees in nursing in England. *International Journal Nursing Studies, 28*, 257–265.

Fritsch, K. (1992). South Pacific nursing education: Visions of the future. *International Nursing Review, 39*, 19–20.

Henry, P. R. (1993). Distance learning through audioconferencing. *Nurse Educator, 18*, 23–26.

Hirschfeld, M. J., & Holleran, C. (1992). Challenges to nursing from the World Health Organization and the International Council of nurses. *Nursing Administration Quarterly, 16*, 1–3.

Innes, J., & Oulton, J. (1990). Nursing educational goals for the 21st century: Canada. In C. Fagin (Ed.), *Nursing Leadership: Global Strategies* (pp. 67–74). New York: (National League for Nursing Publication No. 41–2349).

King, J. (1988). Differences between RN and generic students and the impact on the educational process. *Journal of Nursing Education, 27*, 131–135.

Knowles, M. S. (1980). *The modern practice of adult education: From pedagogy to andragogy*. Chicago: Association Press/Follett.

Lengacher, C., & Van Cott, M. R. (1992). Nursing research related to educational re-entry for the registered nurse. In L. Allen (Ed.), *Review of Research in Nursing Education* New York: (National League for Nursing Publication No. 15–2448).

Lethbridge, D. (1989). Motivational orientations of registered nurse baccalaureate students in rural New England. *Journal of Nursing Education, 28*, 203–208.

Lorensen, M., & Schei, B. (1992). Higher education via satellite. *International Nursing Review, 39*, 5.

MacLean, T., Knoll, G., & Kinney, C. (1985). The evolution of a baccalaureate program for registered nurses. *Journal of Nursing Education, 24*, 53–57.

Marquis, B. J., Lillibridge, J., & Madison, J. (1993). Problems and progress as Australia adopts the bachelor's degree as the only entry to nursing practice. *Nursing Outlook, 41*, 135–140.

Mattson, S. (1990). Coping and developmental maturity of RN baccalaureate students. *Western Journal of Nursing Research, 12*, 514–524.

McHugh, M. (1991). Direct articulation of AD nursing students into an RN-to-BSN completion program: A research study. *Journal of Nursing Education, 30*, 293–296.

Merritt, S. (1983). Learning style preferences of baccalaureate nursing students. *Nursing Research, 32*, 367–372.

Osei-Boateng, B. (1992). Nursing in Africa today. *International Nursing Review, 39*, 175–180.

Paulanka, B. J. (1993). Distance education for RN students. In Diekelman, N. L., & Rather, M. L., (Eds.), *Transforming RN education: Dialogue and debate* (pp. 324–338). Newark, DE: (National League for Nursing Publication No. 14–2511).

Ryan, M. (1985). Assimilating the learning needs of RN students into the clinical practicum. *Journal of Nursing Education, 24*, 128–130.

Shomaker, D. (1993). A statewide instructional television program via satellite for RN-to-BSN students. *Journal of Professional Nursing, 9*, 153–8.

Thompson, C. (1992). Nontraditional students in higher education: A review of the literature and implications for nursing education. In L. Allen (Ed.), *Review of Research in nursing Education* (Vol. 5) (pp. 31–43). New York: (National League for Nursing Publication No. 15–2448).

Thurber, F. (1988). A comparison of RN students in two types of baccalaureate completion programs. *Journal of Nursing Education, 27*, 266–273.

Woodman, E., Knecht, L., Periard, M., & Bell, E. (1991). Assessment of affective outcomes in RN/BSN Programs: Advancing Toward professionalism. In M. Garbin (Ed.), *Educational outcomes*. New York: (National League for Nursing Publication No. 15–247).

World Health Organization. (1978). *Report of the International Conference on Primary Health Care: Alma-Ata, USSR*. Geneva: Author.

CHAPTER 17

Organizational Aspects of Nursing Education from a Global Perspective

Irmajean Bajnok, RN, PhD

W hen exploring organizational aspects of nursing education, it is imperative to acknowledge that nursing education is a part of the broad culture and context of the environment. Education is a reflection of social, political, economical, and technical realities within a culture. To understand the organizational aspects of nursing education on a global perspective, it is necessary to appreciate the culture and context of the setting.

Some aspects may be in existence, may be possible, or impossible in some countries because of the political situation, cultural norms, or economic realities. To comprehend what is happening in nursing education, then, it is important to see it in the context of the totality of the country. This chapter will share a model for understanding the organizational aspects of nursing education from the perspectives of social, political, economical, technical and cultural realities.

What is meant by organizational aspects of nursing education? Six elements are considered as significant organizational aspects of nursing programs. They are:

- mission and philosophy;
- academic leadership;
- organizational infrastructure;
- standards, policies and procedures;
- strategic planning; and
- resources, material and human.

THE MISSION AND PHILOSOPHY

Mission and philosophy addresses the overall purpose of the educational unit, and the values and beliefs that will direct the achievement of that purpose (Swansburg, 1990). Mission and philosophy include such aspects as the

151

focus of the faculty on teaching, research, and/or practice, and the focus of the curriculum on health promotion, illness care, or both. They also incorporate the relationships with service, with other health professionals, and with those "outside" health care. Finally, the nature of candidates who are recruited as students and faculty and how recruitment is carried out also are influenced by philosophy and mission. In fact the mission and philosophy will have an impact on all the other organizational aspects. Mission and philosophy may be explicit in a written statement, or they may be implicit, evident only through the other organizational aspects.

ACADEMIC LEADERSHIP

Academic leadership incorporates such issues as: Who leads the academic unit—is it nursing, medicine, or some other discipline? What type of leadership is it? Is it autocratic leadership, or a more academic/democratic model of leadership? How is the leadership determined? Is the academic leadership congruent with the mission and philosophy? What impact does the academic leadership have vis-á-vis the mission and philosophy?

ORGANIZATIONAL INFRASTRUCTURE

Organizational infrastructure is a broad area that includes reporting structures, committee structures, scope of decisionmaking of students, faculty, and administration, and who has final authority.

STANDARDS, POLICIES, AND PROCEDURES

Standards, policies, and procedures all act as guides to administration, faculty, and students as they seek to achieve the mission and philosophy through the organizational infrastructure.

STRATEGIC PLANNING

Strategic planning is a process by which systems examine the past, present, and future trends in order to have the most relevant and effective system possible (Quinn, Faerman, Thompson, & McGrath, 1990; Swansburg, 1990). In educational institutions curriculum planning incorporates strategic planning processes.

RESOURCES, MATERIAL AND HUMAN . . . INCLUDING FACULTY, STUDENTS, PATIENTS, PRACTICING NURSES, OTHER HEALTH CARE WORKERS, AND OTHERS

In this area it is important to note what and who are considered resources in a school of nursing. Some schools will consider only the more traditional material and human resources. Others will focus on nurses, a variety of health care professionals, scientists, researchers, and lawyers, among others, as human resources. They will also include a diversity of health care settings as material resources.

To understand how these organizational aspects are shaped and how they influence education, it is important to examine them in light of the relevant political, social, economical, technical, and cultural forces. Five themes have been selected for discussion that illustrate the interrelationship of organizational aspects and the above-mentioned forces. The themes are examined as to their importance in nursing education in various countries; why they are important in light of the forces identified; and how they have influenced the organizational aspects. The five themes are:

1) Gender and nursing;
2) Health promotion;
3) The changing curriculum;
4) Service/education collaboration; and
5) Entry-level education.

The examination of each theme will indicate which sociocultural-technical forces are involved and which organizational aspects of nursing education have been influenced. Also noted will be where these themes differ internationally and why.

GENDER AND NURSING

Globally, nursing is a female-dominated profession. Just how female-dominated varies from country to country. For example, countries in Eastern Europe and England have more males in nursing than Canada, the United States, and many South American and Asian countries. However, the sociocultural notions of the role of women have influenced, and continue to influence, nursing and nursing education (Larsen & Baumgart, 1992). All nurses have been affected by the "taboo on knowledge" which relegated to women a short, more practical type of education because they were not seen to be suited to the rigors of serious study (Gillett, 1981). Witness the fact that in

Canada it has only been in the last 10 to 15 years that education for nurses has been primarily in the general education system. The move of nursing education to the general education system brought with it standards, policies, and procedures more similar to other post-secondary educational programs, and changes in academic leadership (Larsen & Baumgart, 1992). In particular, there has been a move to a more collegial and democratic type of leadership.

In some countries in Europe and Asia, nursing education has been and still is part of secondary education. In many instances this has barred nurses from university education, which has created a major barrier for many women to advance their education. Of course this has had an impact on academic leadership and the organizational infrastructure in schools of nursing. Nurses without advanced preparation could hardly be expected to take on leadership roles in educational institutions. Therefore, in many countries, male physicians have taken on this role.

Slowly, in many countries, as it becomes socially, politically, and economically expedient to recognize women as equal to men, the knowledge taboo for women is lifting. However, this has not meant that nursing has moved into the universities, attracting the best and the brightest male and female students (Larsen & Baumgart, 1992a and b). Socially, in the West and many other countries, nursing is still associated with a negative stereotype of being women's work and a role that does not offer much power, status, or control (Muff, 1982). Therefore, large numbers of men are not enrolling in nursing and indeed, more women are enrolling in those professions that are perceived to have more status than nursing (Larsen & Baumgart, 1992). This has influenced strategic planning, and standards, policies, and procedures related to student recruitment, promotion, and attrition in schools of nursing.

In many countries, particularly South America, Europe, and Asia, the social status afforded physicians has meant that the number of physicians per 1000 population is disproportionately high in relation to the number of nurses per 1000 population. Even with economic and political forces at work, this phenomenon will take a long time to change, and its impact on organizational aspects of nursing education will be apparent well into the new millennium.

HEALTH PROMOTION

For a long time acute illness care and technology for diagnosis and treatment have dominated the health care agenda. This has influenced the mission and philosophy of nursing education, types of resources, and standards, policies, and procedures.

As it becomes clear to policymakers that, economically and politically, health care reform must focus on primary health care and health promotion, more resources are being diverted to these areas (World Bank, 1993). This is beginning to happen in North and South America, some countries in Eastern Europe, and the West Indies. Other countries are reviving their outpost health stations and reemphasizing primary health care. In these countries, changes in nursing education have led to a greater focus on health promotion, independent outpost practice, and community participation. Curriculum resources have broadened to include the family, community groups, polyclinics, and settings where health promotion is experienced.

As more questions are asked related to what keeps people healthy, and at what cost, there is more interest in faculty who can contribute to health care reform through research on health promotion. Thus, for economic reasons, research on health promotion and care verses cure is becoming more valued. While this is happening to a great degree in the Western world, it is also a factor in Eastern and Western Europe, where illness care is seen as costing too much and having too little impact on the standard of living and health for all.

THE CHANGING CURRICULUM

Expression of the need for curriculum change seems to be a phenomenon of nursing education in many countries (Baumgart & Larsen, 1992; Salvage, 1993). Nursing education in North America in the past was focused on the curriculum as planning, teaching and evaluating theory "for" nursing to the exclusion of focusing on teaching the understanding and application of theory "of" nursing. This orientation no doubt was attributable to the large numbers of nurse faculty who had received graduate preparation in programs which were focused on education and curriculum development rather than on nursing (Meleis, 1985). It also was influenced by the fact that nursing theory was in its early developmental stages. The increase in the numbers of nurses with advanced preparation in nursing and research has fostered the nursing theory movement and the development of a more balanced curricular focus on theory, theory-based practice and research. Resources in schools or nursing are beginning to reflect this change (Larsen & Baumgart, 1992). As well, standards, policies, and procedures acknowledge the importance of both acquisition of knowledge and the ability to apply this knowledge in practice. In addition, clinical practice is expected to be based on theory.

There is a general understanding globally that in a practice discipline, clinical education is as important as theory and must be integrated with theory. In some countries in South America, and Europe this is just beginning to be emphasized (Salvage, 1993). In other countries, such as China, there has not been as much of a social or cultural push for these changes.

The focus on health promotion and the increase in technology have both had an impact on organizational aspects of nursing education. Advances in knowledge and technology have meant that nurses in many countries are carrying out functions that used to be the domain of physicians and medicine. In turn, nursing education has become more complex.

Nursing education programs must engage in strategic planning to determine how best to structure curricula with a balance of illness- and health-oriented content; theory and practice; generalist and specialist content; and a reflection of demographic trends (Larsen & Baumgart, 1992; Williams, 1992). Planning activities must also be focused on determining what are appropriate resources as well as on plans for their acquisition and use. However, in some countries, where social forces dictate that technology represents status, there is a continuing focus on increasing this content in the curriculum to the exclusion of health promotion and primary health care content.

Technological advances also have created changes in modes of curriculum delivery in order to accommodate a variety of forms of distance education. Economic and political forces have influenced developments in this area as well. For many countries this has meant or could mean that basic, continuing, and advanced education are much more accessible. Advances in technology have had an impact on the mission and philosophy of nursing education, the organizational infrastructure, material and human resources (especially the student resource, given distance education), strategic planning, and standards, policies, and procedures.

SERVICE EDUCATION COLLABORATION

Because of nursing education's early focus on the "doing" rather than on the "thinking" aspects of nursing, and because of the sociocultural views of education for women, there was not a perceived service/education rift in the past (Larsen & Baumgart, 1992). In other words, since there was only service and a "doing" mentality, there was no basis for a rift.

In many countries, the move to upgrade the educational preparation for nurses has brought with it an initial devaluing of the practice of nursing and a movement of nurses away from patient care and the clinical aspects of nursing. In those countries now embarking on upgrading educational preparation, this phenomenon could be avoided if attention is paid to history and the negative side effects of focusing on theory to the exclusion of practice.

Social and economic realities are moving nursing service and education back together. Socially, it is becoming clear that the clinical skills of nurses, whether used in health or illness situations, are what is unique about nursing (Yura-Petro & Brooks, 1991). Nurses do not practice, educate, research, or administer in a vacuum. Clinical nurses provide nursing interventions related to patient needs. Nurse faculty teach nursing knowledge and skills and their application in practice settings. Nurse researchers carry out research to develop the discipline of nursing, and nurse administrators provide leadership and management in the provision of nursing care. This view has influenced the types of resources needed in education programs as practice settings are welcomed as partners, expert clinicians are jointly appointed to universities, and nurses with higher education in nursing, clinical specialties, and research are recruited to faculties (Holden-Lund, Tate, & Hyde-Robertson, 1991; Kirkpatrick, Byrne, Martin, & Roth, 1991).

Economical forces have also been an impetus for education/service collaboration in some countries. In the West, in particular, as health and education budgets are reduced, both service and education see collaboration as having mutual financial benefits (Redman, Bednash, & Amos, 1990). Service agencies with many student placements are able to realize some cost saving in care provision, and can save on staff recruitment and orientation costs.

Academic institutions are collaborating with service to offer clinical appointments to nursing staff who act as preceptors and role models for nursing students. This relieves faculty to take on more of a facilitator role to both students and staff, and to have more time for clinical collaborative research activities (Dufault, Bartlett, Dagrosa, & Dayle, 1992; Infante, Forbes, Houldin, & Naylor, 1989; Stark & Dison, 1987). This has simulated changes in organizational infrastructure as roles are created for clinical associates, as joint appointments are recognized, and as reporting relationships integrate service and educational institutions. Unification models in nursing education represent major infrastructure and academic leadership change as administrators and faculty take on both service and education roles (Yarcheski & Mahon, 1985, 1986). Education/service collaboration has also effected changes in mission and philosophy; standards, policies, and procedures; and resources.

ENTRY-LEVEL EDUCATION

It is apparent that in most parts of the world social, cultural, and technical forces have altered views of what the entry level of nursing education should be. Generally there is some agreement among nurses, health care providers, and the public that the entry level should be advanced beyond what it currently is. Therefore, in countries where nursing education has been part of secondary education, there is agreement that it should be at the postsecondary level, and many European countries are moving rapidly in this direction (Salvage, 1993). Where nursing education has been at a postsecondary level, again there is some agreement that it should be at a university level (Bajnok, 1992). An alteration of the entry level of education clearly has an impact on all the organizational aspects of nursing education. A change of this magnitude takes much planning and sensitivity to the forces involved.

The impact of professional forces as a factor in organizational aspects of nursing education, while not addressed as a theme, warrants some mention here. It is suggested that professional forces operate in two ways. First, the organized professional may work to create a major social force for change. This strategy is very hard to accomplish unless the issue is broad enough to involve other interest groups. Second, the organized profession may take advantage of a major social force for change and work to make relevant changes in the profession. This strategy is easier to carry out, but still requires much skill, especially in initially recognizing the window of opportunity and being prepared for it. In the latter case the organized profession provides direction and substance to the change. In fact, in many of the themes outlined in this paper, the organized nursing profession was able to take advantage of the opportunity and undertake the necessary action to create and shape the changes in nursing education.

In summary, the thesis of this chapter has been that organizational aspects of nursing education, which include mission and philosophy; academic leadership; organizational infrastructure; standards, policies, and procedures; strategic planning; and resources, are influenced by social, political, economic, technical, and cultural forces. These forces differ in many instances from country to country. Understanding organizational aspects of nursing education from a global perspective means being sensitive to the sociocultural, economical and technical context within a country. Perhaps the sharing of education research in international conferences and meetings and the resulting globalization of nursing education will enhance how all nurse educators create and respond to sociocultural forces in the future.

REFERENCES

Bajnok, I. (1992). Entry level educational preparation for nurses. In A. Baumgart & J. Larsen, (Eds.), *Canadian nursing faces the future* (pp. 401–419). Toronto: Mosby Year Book.

Baumgart, A., & Larsen, J. (Eds.) (1992). *Canadian nursing faces the future*. Toronto: Mosby Year Book.

Dufault, M., Bartlett, B., Dagrosa, C., & Dayle, J. (1992). A statewide consortium initiative to establish an undergraduate clinical internship program. *Journal of Professional Nursing, 8,* 239–244.

Gillett, M. (1981). *We walked very warily*. Montreal: Eden Press Women's Publications.

Holden-Lund, C., Tate, E., & Hyde-Robertson, B. (1991). Consortium model for master's education in nursing, *Nurse Educator, 16,* 13–17.

Infante, M. S., Forbes, E., Houldin, A., & Naylor, M. (1989). A clinical teaching: Examination of a clinical teaching model. *Journal of Professional Nursing, 5,* 132–139.

Kirkpatrick, H., Byrne, C., Martin, M. L. & Roth, M. L. (1991). A collaborative model for the clinical education of baccalaureate nursing students. *Journal of Advanced Nursing, 16,* 101–107.

Larsen, J. & Baumgart, A. (1992). Overview: Issues in nursing education. In A. Baumgart & J. Larsen (Eds.), *Canadian nursing faces the future* (pp. 383–400). Toronto: Mosby Year Book.

Meleis, A. (1985). *Theoretical nursing: Development and progress.* Philadelphia: Lippincott.

Muff, J. (1982). *Socialization, sexism, and stereotyping: Women's issues in nursing.* St. Louis: Mosby.

Quinn, R., Faerman, S., Thompson, M., & McGrath, M. (1990). *Becoming a master manager: A competency framework.* New York: Wiley.

Redman, B., Bednash, G., & Amos, L. (1990). Policy perspectives on economic investment in professional nursing education. *Nursing Economics, 8,* 27–35.

Salvage, J. (Ed.), (1993). *Nursing in action: Strengthening nursing and midwifery to support health for all.* (European Series, No. 48) Copenhagen: WHO Regional Publications.

Swansburg, R. (1990). *Management and leadership for nurse managers.* Boston: Jones & Bartlett.

Stark, J., & Dison, C. (1987). A model linking education and practice. *Journal of Nursing Staff Development, 3,* 24–27.

World Bank. (1993). *World development report, 1993: Investing in health.* Oxford: Oxford University Press.

Williams, G. (1992). Nursing education in New Zealand. *International Nursing Review, 39,* 21–23.

Yarcheski, A., & Mahon, N. (1985). The unification model in nursing: A study of receptivity among nurse educators in the United States. *Nursing Research, 34,* 120–125.

Yarcheski, A., & Mahon, N. (1986). The unification model in nursing: Risk-receptivity profiles among deans, tenured, and nontenured faculty in the United States. *Western Journal of Nursing Research, 8,* 63–81.

Yura-Petro, H., & Brooks, J. (1991). Congruence between nursing education and nursing service: A common conceptual/theoretical framework for nursing units. *The Health Care Supervisory, 10,* 1–12.

PART IV

Advancing Research in Nursing Education

CHAPTER 18

Pathways to Implementing Nursing Education Research Globally

Joyce J. Fitzpatrick, RN, MBA, PhD, FAAN

Health care for the citizens of the world is an important component of our increasingly complex global economies. Worldwide, nurses comprise the greatest health care resource, not only in quantity, but also in quality. As front line providers of primary, secondary, and tertiary health care services, nurses are in a strategic position to influence the future.

The future of the profession, and, some might say, the health care of the world population, lies in the hands, the hearts, and the heads of the nurse educators, for theirs is the challenge of preparing the next generation of health care providers. Nurse educators today must prepare the nurses of the future to care for the people of today and tomorrow.

For too long nursing education and practice have been guided by tradition rather than based on research. More recently, nurse educators have embraced the scientific tradition. International conferences such as the one held in Bolzano, Italy serve as important landmarks in the journey to advance our profession. As we move through this journey, it is important to mark our progress and carry a road map for continuing the journey.

This chapter is an effort to recognize some of our accomplishments in nursing education and nursing education research, some of the landmarks that are important in our history, that serve as exemplars of the progress that we have made. In addition, a pathway to the future will be outlined. It is the hope that together nurses may pool their expertise and resources, set aside our twentieth-century modes of transportation through the path of nursing education, and move rapidly into the twenty-first century.

EXEMPLARS IN NURSING EDUCATION AND ITS RESEARCH

Visionary leadership in nursing education is evident across international boundaries, from the Project 2000 initiatives in the U.K., to the new "distance learning" models in Zimbabwe, from the requirement for nursing informatics in some programs in the United States for basic students, to the re-emphasis of basic nursing skills, from the experiments in nursing, both formal and informal, that brought nursing education and service environments closer together, from the high tech, high touch models of nursing to philosophical and conceptual models that serve as the fabric for development of educational programs. Revolutionaries in nursing education research are in every country, struggling and thriving at the same time. It is important to celebrate educational successes to avoid discouragement and fatigue from the daily challenges, and to avoid losing sight of the longer-term goals.

When we launched the landmark *Annual Review of Nursing Research* series in 1983, Dr. Harriet Werley and I made a formal commitment to include at least one chapter per volume focused on nursing education research. We also made a commitment to include chapters detailing the status of nursing research in other countries besides our own. What we have discovered in the past decade is that there is a thirst for knowledge on nursing education research and there is an expressed interest in more of an international focus in our work. Researchers consistently report that these critical review chapters serve as an important starting point for their own review of the literature, guiding their research to a more substantive question, raising and clarifying issues that lead them to a sounder study.

We have commissioned chapters from many countries and we are particularly interested in ascertaining the nursing education research that has been done historically either in one country or across national groupings, e.g., South America, Eastern Europe. We look forward to the expansion of our international focus in this ARNR series.

PATHWAY TO THE FUTURE

As we move forward to advance nursing education research, both individual and collective actions are necessary on the part of nurse educators and researchers. Through a community of scholarship we expect to achieve results which demonstrate that the "whole is greater than the sum of the parts." We can use others' research as a springboard for our own scholarship and we can share resources, both personal and financial.

Individual Action

Three characteristics of individual action will be discussed. These include competence, communication, and commitment. If you remember nothing else from this chapter, remember these key concepts, for they form the foundation for both individual and collective action in our pursuit of excellence in our discipline.

Competence

We must prepare ourselves with the requisite knowledge for active research in our discipline. For some of us that will require a formal program of educational study; for some, continuing education in targeted areas will be necessary; and others can best prepare themselves through self-study. We must continue our curiosity about the potential for advances in our content, our teaching methods, and our outcome evaluations. And, importantly, we must actively seek the support and involvement of others, particularly scientists in other disciplines, through collegial exchanges, and informal and formal collaborative interdisciplinary research.

Communication

Our scholarship is not complete without the final act of communication and dissemination. While the traditional ways of formal scientific communication are known to all of us, i.e., publications and presentations at scientific sessions, we do not yet have a tradition of scholarship within our profession. It is time to build that important tradition, to construct a firm foundation for future generations of nurse researchers and nurse educators. Our strength will be based on the firmest foundation that we can possibly construct. There are some very simple activities that can influence our individual and collective expertise.

1) We can read scholarly journals in nursing;

2) We can exchange ideas with each other. For example, the next time you read an interesting article about an experiment in nursing education be certain to jot a note to the author, sharing your thoughts and creating the opportunity for scholarly dialogue;

3) We can make all of our teaching a research experience, but introducing, at a minimum, a systematic evaluation component, and/or a formal outcome-driven research design;

4) We can present and publish our educational research;

5) We can attend conferences, and engage in dialogue with other researchers.

Commitment

If there is one requirement of all of the activities cited above, it is commitment. We must be committed to the necessary discipline and the procedures for change. Our values must be consistent with those of an inquiring mind.

Collective Action

Collective action requires a shared mindset, and most importantly, collaboration. While collaboration is a frequently cited goal, particularly among interdisciplinary health professional groups, it is not a goal that is automatically accomplished only by communication. Collaboration requires an overlap in goals, and a commitment to work toward common interests to achieve desired outcomes that are mutually beneficial. Collaboration requires work!

Collaborative transcultural research

We can learn much from the crosscultural collaborative clinical nursing research that has become more prominent in the past decade. And we can begin to design our educational programs so that we build together, to determine both the similarities and the differences within our profession across our national and continental boundaries. We can begin to answer important questions such as: Will a primary care orientation in a basic nursing curriculum be as effective in meeting the health care needs of the citizens of California as those in Portugal? What are the short-term and long-term needs for nurses in primary care in each of our countries, and how can we best design educational programs to respond to the pressing demands?

Formal university and/or interinstitutional affiliation agreements

Many of our institutions have existing relationships based on shared expertise and/or interest in basic sciences, the humanities, the arts, and medical science. The general format of the formal affiliation agreement, which often constitutes a legal contract, consists of a statement of shared mission and goals, with more specific statements about that which will be committed by each participating institution. Specific components might include faculty and student exchange, and formal collaborative research between the institutions, shared resources such as library resources, conference planning, etc.

Sister city relationships

In a world of changing and developing world economies, many of our cities have developed ''sister city'' relationships with cities where there is a common economic interest, often linked by cultural ties. In circumstances where these relationships exist, we should build collaborative nursing educational relationships upon existing formal relationships.

CALL TO CITIZENSHIP

As we advance our disciplinary knowledge, each and all of us must be called to citizenship in the global nursing education research community. We have taken giant steps in convening and participating in the Bolzano conference, but this is only the beginning of our journey. We must fortify ourselves with knowledge and gather all of the tools that might be necessary in order to thrive on this important trip.

CHAPTER 19

A Blueprint for Advancing Nursing Education Research Globally

Scientific Committee Members *

E ducation will play an essential role in building nursing's future. It is critical to the preparation of professionals as clinical nurses, managers, educators, and researchers all over the world, and ultimately in the improvement of the quality of care that nurses provide their patients/clients. As the world itself is changing and becoming more interrelated, nursing education must assume an increasingly international perspective. Therefore, nurse educators need to continually examine and develop existing content and introduce new goals, content, and teaching methods to meet the health care needs of the people they serve.

One important way to develop new programs and instruments is through research. The international conference on Expanding Boundaries of Nursing Education Globally (held in October 1993 at Bolzano, Italy) has stressed the need for an increase in research on nursing education. Through this document, emerging from the suggestions of all the presenters at the Conference and from several deliberations among the Committee members, the Scientific Committee of the Conference offers a contribution to the topic. The document is presented as a framework for the future. Key issues are identified, with particular attention to bridging the current gaps in research knowledge, and importantly, setting the stage for future collaboration globally. Also, it was our belief that by highlighting our successes through this Conference, we could identify our goals and build a foundation for the future.

We hope that this document will serve as a basis for discussion in many educational and research settings and a stimulus to everyone to cooperate in undertaking and developing research projects in nursing education.

This document reports elements referring to:

*Margaret Alexander (Scotland), Irmajean Bajnok (Canada), Colleen Conway-Welch (USA), Joyce J. Fitzpatrick (USA), Kornelia Helembai (Hungary), Brigitta Hochnegger-Haubmann (Austria), Zeinab Loutfi (Egypt), Geraldine McCarthy (Ireland), Diane McGivern (USA), Doris Modly (USA), Mary Mundinger (USA), Piera Poletti (Italy), Sheila Ryan (USA), Jane Salvage (Denmark), Majda Slajmer-Japelj (Slovenia), Marta Stankova (Czech Republic), Marianne Tallberg (Finland), Konrad Tratter (Italy) and Renzo Zanotti (Italy)

1) Significant areas for development in nursing education;
2) Targeted areas for nursing education research;
3) Recommendations regarding research methods and instruments;
4) Advancement of research roles, responsibilities, and sites;
5) Policies to be pursued at local, regional, national, and international levels;
6) Avenues of funding;
7) Recommended strategies.

1. Significant Areas for Development in Nursing Education

Research has to be initiated to address nursing education problems where there is a lack of knowledge. The Committee has identified a list of problems to serve as an impetus for research in the field. Significant areas for development include:

- Recognize the contributions of nursing to society, leading to resources and support, especially through funding for nursing education, basic, postbasic, and continuing education;
- Enhance the quality of nursing education, recognizing the differences in the standards and quality of nursing education around the world;
- Develop and test innovative teaching models in classroom and clinical settings; evaluate the current models of teaching in relation to quality outcomes and effectiveness; enhance the ability of academic and clinical staff to influence student learning; develop model clinical staff for students to emulate;
- Enhance the clinical skills of faculty/nurse educators and the teaching of clinical judgment;
- Evaluate nursing conceptualizations for their curricular relevance with specific attention to the application of theory to practice in clinical settings (e.g., hospitals, homes, community agencies) and the classroom;
- Focus teacher career planning on teacher preparation, including both clinical competencies and research training, and commitment to teaching as a career;
- Define the advantages of educational systems for nursing education and develop new models, including the organizational aspects of the nursing schools;
- Develop community-based models of education that include attention to collaborative relationships with families and communities;
- Enhance awareness among nurse educators of the need for research in nursing education for advancing the knowledge of the discipline; em-

phasize the specific role of nurse educators in supporting research on nursing education;

- Evaluate current models for curricula development, including attention to essential content and priorities for satisfying legal requirements and professional needs;
- Strengthen the service and education interface in order to increase the research/practice link to educate for the future needs of society;
- Evaluate components of nursing education focused on primary health care goals;
- Assess the interface of nursing education with education of other health professionals; evaluate changes in nursing and effects on other health professionals;
- Evaluate the social isolation of nursing students in some programs in some countries and the value of broader university-based education;
- Assess continuing education needs of professional nurses for lifelong learning; and
- Develop models for continuing education teaching/learning.

2. Targeted Areas for Nursing Education Research

Referring to the most urgent problems in a worldwide perspective, the areas identified as priorities for research are the following:

- Prerequisites for admission into nursing education programs and selection procedures;
- Relationship between level of nursing education and health outcomes;
- Methods for educating for interpersonal relationships; use of interpersonal relationships; development of communication and collaboration skills with patients/clients, families, and other health professionals;
- Evaluation of alternative clinical and laboratory settings for nursing education beyond traditional hospital settings, with particular attention to settings for primary care;
- Evaluation of interface between teaching methods and student learning;
- Evaluation of ways to teach values and ethics, and influence the affective domain;
- Criteria for evaluating student learning of various skills and ways of knowing;
- Methods of assisting students at advanced levels to assume aspects of the professional role, reflecting service, education, research, and administration;
- Evaluation of models for general and specialty education in nursing and

their impact on the teacher role; evaluation of the effects of the education model on nursing practice;

- Educational needs of advanced practitioners in nursing and educational models for their preparation; assessment of continuing education needs and methods;
- Methods of teacher preparation, including the teaching of research at all levels within nursing education;
- Methods and tools for conducting nursing education research; with particular attention to the international or crosscultural dimensions;
- Experiments with the use of different forms of information technology to support effectiveness and efficiency of nursing education;
- Identification of methods to improve the use of information technology to support nursing education research; and
- Development of models for research on re-entry education and model programs for re-entering students.

3. Recommendations Regarding Research Methods and Instruments

The development of nursing in all the world's countries is producing patterns of knowledge with some common features. However, some potential innovations for nursing education still remain at local levels and have no diffusion outside the countries' borders. The dialectics among cultural diversities and national customs could be an important approach to improving the standards of nursing education in the next decade. Multisite, replication, and crosscultural research permits increases in the generalization of scientific findings and, at the same time, reduces national diversities. Thus, the transferability of research findings to practice in different cultural settings needs to be better explored. Multinational collaboration on nursing education research should be one of the most important goals for the near future.

The Committee recommends an eclectic approach to research. Therefore, a wide range of research methods has to be used, according to the phenomena to be studied. Both quantitative and qualitative methods are recommended to achieve integration between them. In some complex research projects, triangulation can be useful. Referring to some of the points cited as trends, some examples are given in order to stress the importance of the different methods. In order to describe specific national educational models and their peculiarities, historical research can be useful. Through such study, one can find out which circumstances and events in the past have influenced nursing education. In a cognitive sense, history can be used for predicting the future. And studies on earlier methods to teach nursing skills could, perhaps, reveal long-forgotten useful techniques.

In countries with multiethnic populations, nursing schools must become more culturally diverse in their student and faculty composition. Cross-cultural comparative research and ethnographic research also have to be supported to explore cultural attitudes and values and their impact on the educational process. Much effort needs to be devoted to inquiry into the development and impact of the intrinsic didactic act in different settings and circumstances; experimental and quasi-experimental methods are mostly required for this purpose. Finally, in research projects, attention has to be given to the methods themselves, to better understand their potential in the educational research field and, perhaps, find new ones. Critical review of the literature, including meta-analysis, has to be increased.

The aim of all education, including nursing education, is to provide knowledge and influence change of human behavior in a specific direction. In the case of nursing education, the aim is behavior exhibited by the learner that is congruous with behavior expected of a person providing nursing care in the context of a particular health care setting. Since outcomes of education are reflected in human behavior, the methods used to study a system of nursing education, its processes and outcomes, as well as the concepts important to nursing education, will therefore be based on data reflected in the behavior of the learner (student or practicing nurse) and the teacher of nursing. Tools for the study of their behavior, both verbal and nonverbal, can be grouped into interactional research tools and tools that use nonverbal techniques for the collection of data.

Interactional research tools are based on interactions between the researcher and subjects, direct verbalization or via a questionnaire, and thus are "ideational" and considered more intrusive than the nonverbal techniques of participant and nonparticipant observation, historical research, record reviews, etc. Various alternative nonverbal techniques exist for observing relevant phenomena in nursing education. The suggested tools are not a complete inventory. The researcher, therefore, should constantly be alert to the possibilities of developing new modes of collecting relevant data that best answer the research questions. Examples of instruments that could be used include questionnaires, observation, checklists, interview schedules, and diaries. Particular attention must be paid to the validity and form of the instruments, because these are used in different cultural groups.

4. Advancement of Research Roles, Responsibilities, and Sites

Even if the development of education is the ethical responsibility of every nurse, people directly involved in the field have a greater investment in its advancement. The single faculty member and the researcher have additional responsibilities beyond carrying out their own research projects, teaching from a research basis, and expecting students to reflect a research-based practice.

The nurse educators must also promote research on education and stimulate subjects and institutions to fund research.

Professional organizations are expected to put as much energy as possible into promoting this specific kind of research, because investing in the future of education is the main road to improving nursing service and, consequently, the status of nursing in society and the recognition of nurses' contributions to health.

The most appropriate settings for promoting, organizing, and managing educational research are universities/institutions of higher education and research institutes. They can provide methodological expertise and appropriate technical resources to be used in the projects. In addition, they can have a broader view than one of just a single phenomenon and can develop research project networks.

Sites for carrying out research include all traditional and current educational settings and potential new sites; the following are just a few examples: classrooms, skills laboratories, clinical placement areas, patients' homes, and community services.

5. Policies to be Pursued at Local, Regional, National, and International Levels

In order to increase the attention paid to the issue it is proposed that recommendations be advanced at multiple levels within various groups. Nurse educators involved in research can assume the responsibility for raising the level of awareness and delineating specific policies. Individual actions are required, but are not sufficient in themselves. At local, regional, national, and international levels formal policies have to be promoted. Referring to their specific responsibilities, institutions should be strongly encouraged to write resolutions on the issue. The following are presented as examples:

- Resolutions passed by professional organizations (ICN and national associations);
- Official bodies' statements of support; e.g., WHO, Union Council of Europe, and other international organizations with health duties; and
- Individual nations through policy-making bodies.

6. Avenues of Funding

A range of avenues for funding must be explored, including those that have not previously been exposed to such endeavors. It will be paramount that nurse educators determine specific relationships of the research to the goals of potential funding agencies or institutions and, at the same time, influence the priorities of the funding agencies. The following are examples of potential sources of support:

- Health boards/ministries/departments, international and national governmental organizations, nursing associations;
- Multinational corporations, especially those with health interests, including health care technology, pharmaceutical, and computing industries; and
- Foundations (Rockefeller, Kellogg, etc.), family, and charitable foundations.

7. Recommended Strategies

An effort must be made to identify and initiate a multiplicity of strategies. The following are examples of strategies:

- Develop public information campaigns to highlight research findings, inside and outside the professional field;
- Create an information system for sharing progress (telematics);
- Use computers and other technology in order to carry out research and share research (e.g., through electronic mail);
- Develop and/or expand retrieval systems that include nursing classification; e.g., the Metathesaurus of the Unified Medical Language System (UMLS) developed through the National Library of Medicine in the United States;
- Disseminate information regarding research methodologies and findings;
- Develop conferences and other methods of sharing information to exchange ideas and experiences relevant to nursing education research;
- Increase the exchange of research through international nursing journals;
- Submit proposals that have multiple sites and multiple countries involved;
- Strengthen the research component of the curricula at all levels;
- Introduce research in teacher's curriculum to prepare a critical mass of nurse educators who are prepared to teach from a research basis and conduct research; develop continuing-education programs in research for existing teachers; and
- Introduce sessions on nursing education research during research conferences.

CONCLUSIONS

This document is a framework for the future; it will be effective only if nurses will address the cited problems and develop research projects. Many strategies have been identified; it is now up to every nurse, researcher, teacher, faculty, executive, director, and dean of schools of nursing to realize these strategies. There will be many obstacles to achieving these goals. The global context is not an easy one, and the global and national economies present challenges at a time when health demands are increasing and health care delivery is changing. There must be a stronger role for nurses and nursing in the delivery of health care, particularly in relation to primary health care and community-based home care. Education is the most important tool we have; however, its development is strongly connected with research. Therefore, research projects have to be increased.

Looking to the future, we look toward globalization. We must develop not just local or national research projects, but also international projects on nursing education research. International cooperation can value the single experience and enrich the common knowledge. We must be aware of one thing: working together requires specific skills, which include understanding cultural diversity, learning from every approach and experience, and developing an attitude of not just "bringing something to," but also "learning something from." This is the great challenge. Through research in education, nursing worldwide can change, and everyone has to contribute to this change.

People attending the conference at Bolzano, Italy came from 36 countries, and this document incorporates many of their suggestions. We hope that these suggestions will be spread out to more and more people in more and more countries, helping them to start a network of worldwide research cooperation.

Index

Z

Zimbabwe, nursing education,
    21–22

$\boxed{\mathbf{SP}}$ *Springer Publishing Company*

KEY ASPECTS OF CARING FOR THE ACUTELY ILL
Technological Aspects, Patient Education, and Quality of Life

Sandra G. Funk, PhD,
Elizabeth M. Tornquist, MA,
Ruth A. Wiese, MSN, RN, and
Mary T. Champagne, PhD, RN, Editors

This volume offers the latest research findings on key aspects of caring for the acutely ill and provides the clinician with the knowledge and means to enhance practice and improve patient care.

Partial Contents:

Key Aspects of Caring for the Acutely Ill, *K. Dracup* • Managing Technology and Complex Care, *K. Stone* • Patient Education, *C. Lindeman* • Maintaining the Patient's Quality of Life, *C. Cooper* • Caring for the Acutely Ill Child, *B.S. Turner*

Evaluating Research Findings for Practice, *L.R. Cronenwett* • Studies of Developmental Nursing Care for Very Low Birth Weight Infants, *P.T. Becker* • The Utilization of a Cognitive-Behavioral Pain Intervention by Children and Parents, *M.E. Broome et al.* • Interventions to Enhance Maternal and Child Coping with Unplanned Childhood Hospitalization, *B. Mazurek Melnyk*

Minimizing Diagnostic Blood Loss in Critically Ill Patients, *E. Gleason et al.* • Rewarming Postoperative Patients, *M. Giuffre* • Child Visitation in Adult Critical Care Units, *M. Titler et al.* • Effects of a Structured and Collaborative Discharge Planning Program, *K.S. Haddock* • Patients' and Family Members' Perceptions of What Makes Quality Patient Care, *M.R. Lynn & S. Sidani* • Improving Outcomes in Patients with Heart Failure, *M.H. Hawthorne & M.E. Hixon* • Research on Caring for the Acutely Ill: Implications for Practice, *M.T. Champagne & R.A. Wiese*

1995   360pp   0-8261-8580-0   hardcover

536 Broadway, New York, NY 10012-3955 • (212) 431-4370 • Fax (212) 941-7842

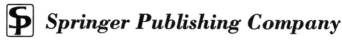

$\boxed{\textbf{SP}}$ *Springer Publishing Company*

ESSENTIALS OF NURSING RESEARCH, 5th Edition

Lucille E. Notter, RN, EdD, FAAN, and
Jacqueline R. Hott, RN, CS, PhD, FAAN

Praise for earlier edition:

"The impressive credentials and rich clinical experience of the authors, combined with their flair for simplifying complex material, enables practice-based scientific inquiry to virtually come alive in these pages ... A winsome 'how-to' manual that will spark the intellectual curiosity and spirit of inquiry in nursing's bright young professionals."

—Nursing Research

Contents:

I. Introduction to Research. Evolution of the Research Movement in Nursing • The Meaning and Purpose of Research

II. The Research Process. Selecting a Problem • The Literature Search • The Hypothesis • The Research Method • Data Collection • Analysis of the Data • Findings, Conclusions, and Recommendations • The Research Report: Communicating the Findings

III. Evaluation of Research. The Evaluation Process

1994   224pp   0-8261-1598-5   softcover

536 Broadway, New York, NY 10012-3955 • (212) 431-4370 • Fax (212) 941-7842

Springer Publishing Company

Annual Review of
Nursing Research, Volume 12
Focus on Significant Clinical Issues

Joyce J. Fitzpatrick, PhD,
Joanne S. Stevenson, PhD, Editors
Nikki S. Polis, PhD, Associate Editor

Now in its second decade of publication, this landmark series draws together and critically reviews all the existing research in specific areas of nursing practice, nursing care delivery, nursing education, and the profession of nursing.

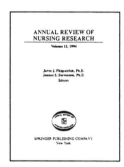

Contents:

1994   264pp   0-8261-8231-3   hardcover

536 Broadway, New York, NY 10012-3955 • (212) 431-4370